W9-BZT-983

Living with Stuttering

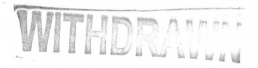

Living with Stuttering

Kenneth O. St. Louis, Ph.D.
Editor

**Stories
Basics
Resources
and Hope**

Populore®

Populore Publishing Company
Morgantown, West Virginia

Triumph Series

Living with Stuttering: Stories, Basics, Resources, and Hope
Kenneth O. St. Louis, Editor

Populore® Publishing Company
PO Box 4382
Morgantown, WV 26504
866-667-8679 orders
304-599-3830 phone
304-599-7224 fax
stories@populore.com
www.populore.com

Design: Angela Caudill
Story Editor: Crystal Hightower

Publisher's Cataloging-in-Publication

Living with stuttering : stories, basics, resources and
   hope / Kenneth O. St. Louis. -- 1st ed.
      p. cm. -- (Triumph series)
      Includes bibliographical references and index.
      LCCN: 2001091798
      ISBN: 0-9652699-4-9

   1. Stuttering--Popular works.   I. St. Louis,
Kenneth O.

   RC424.L58 2001   616.85'54
                               QBI01-200801

Populore books are available at special quantity discounts for bulk purchases for premiums, fund-raising, and educational needs. Reprints of stories, special books, or book excerpts can also be created to fit specific needs. The Taking Stock materials and information found in *Appendices G* and *H* are packaged and available individually. For details, contact the publisher.

Each narrative in *Chapter 2: Our Stories* has been assigned an identification code. The code is found at the end of the narrative with the following six components: Narrative Number-Country-Series (General)-Series (Specific)-Volume Number-Year. For example, the first narrative by Tiffany D. Summerlin is coded 401-001-TR-ST-001-2001. Individual stories will be stored in the Populore Database according to Narrative Numbers, e.g., "No. 401" for Tiffany Summerlin's narrative. Requests for story reprints should include the author's name and the three-digit narrative number.

Reference to any narratives from *Living with Stuttering: Stories, Basics, Resources, and Hope* in other works should cite the author and year within the text, e.g., (Summerlin, 2001). Footnotes, end notes, and/or bibliographic references should include author, year, narrative title, narrative number, author, book title, publisher, and page(s). For example: Summerlin, Tiffany D. 2001. Working Now for a New Attitude. Narrative No. 401. In Kenneth O. St. Louis. *Living with Stuttering: Stories, Basics, Resources, and Hope*. Morgantown, WV: Populore Publishing Company, pp. 31-35.

Printed and bound in the United States of America.

Appendix F: Terminology Pertaining to Fluency and Fluency Disorders: Guidelines. pp. 211 - 218. Reprinted with permission: American Speech-Language-Hearing Association.

To six extraordinary teachers:

Laura Lee Dodd (1st grade), Aunt Grace St.Louis (2nd - 6th grade), Gertrude Campbell (high school), Carl Romano (high school), Bill Leith (undergraduate), and James Jenkins (graduate).

Acknowledgments

I have several birthday cards on my office door that were sent to me over the years by John Ahlbach, current Co-Director of Friends (an organization for young people who stutter) and former Director of the National Stuttering Association, then known as the National Stuttering Project. One card quotes Chesterton, saying, "We are all in the same boat, in a stormy sea, and we owe each other a terrible loyalty." That is especially true for me as it relates to my own story of stuttering and the evolution of this book. I could not have accomplished what I have without the help and support of my family. Rae Jean, who is my best friend and wife—but also the Project Manager for this book and President of Populore Publishing Company—has patiently supported and helped me through challenges with students, stuttering support group meetings, paper revisions, travel, long hours at work, and—yes—even through the stuttering that I still experience. She understands what I do, and I can think aloud and explore ideas with her as well as benefit from her editorial eye, speech-language and linguistics background, and growing expertise in personal history and "stories." My daughter, Melinda, has had a positive influence on my contributions to the field of stuttering in ways she may not even know. Stuttering runs in families, and when Melinda was two years old, she began to stutter quite severely. This happened when I was trying, unsuccessfully, I regret to report, to get a grant to fund a longitudinal study of stuttering children. Thanks to a combination of influences, Melinda completely recovered with no real memories of stuttering at all. She helped influence my now firm decision to recommend treating young stutterers as early as possible.

Thinking of all those who have supported and positively influenced me, I must highlight my late dad, mom, and Aunt Betty, as well as my sister, Rita, and brother, David, for their ongoing support and wisdom. I would not have achieved what I have accomplished in the area of fluency disorders without the collaborative and personal support of numerous mentors and colleagues. Listing all of them would take an entire page, but I must mention specifically Bill Leith, Florence Myers, Gene Brutten, David Daly, Dick Martin, Dick Curlee, Woody Starkweather, the late Einer Boberg, Klaas Bakker, Scott Yaruss, Bob Quesal, Bobbie Lubker, Lena Rustin, Meg Neilson, Hugo Gregory, Gene Cooper, Herman Peters, John Ahlbach, Michael Sugarman, Jaan Pill, and Dobrinka Georgieva as powerful influences on my career. My colleagues in our Department of Speech Pathology and Audiology have been crucial to my success as well, especially Dennis Ruscello and Norm Lass. I must acknowledge my students who carried out many, many interviews of people who stutter. I would be remiss, however, if I did not mention a few who have been singularly important in helping me in the research that culminated in this book: Cara Honig, Heather Ferree, Anna Novotny, Maria Taffoni, Lee Ann Boyd, Kristin Lennex, Mandi Frederick, Katie Bedford, and Karen Oakes. But, especially, I want to highlight the hard work, dedication, and enthusiasm of Crystal Hightower, who is the Story Editor for most of the individual stories in this book. Publications assistants Jessica McDonald and Gail Bossart provided a variety of first-class and much appreciated help. And, thank you Angela Caudill for sharing your refreshing and distinctive talent and skill as a designer.

Most important of all, I acknowledge the hundreds of individuals who stutter—or their parents—who have trusted me and the students I supervise in our Speech Clinic with their lives and futures. We have helped many—though not all—of them, and I have learned important and powerful lessons from each and every one that I hope can be used to help others in the future.

Preface

Living with Stuttering: Stories, Basics, Resources, and Hope is a book for and about people who stutter as well as those who seek to understand and help them. It puts a human face on a problem that has afflicted untold millions of people through the ages. The stories of twenty-five diverse individuals tell the reader that stuttering is not a simple problem of nervousness, as many believe it to be. They attest to the courage and determination of people living day-to-day with a problem that mysteriously but profoundly affects the most basic of human experiences—conversing and interacting with others. But most importantly, the individual authors share their own unique life stories and how stuttering has colored those stories. Reading their personal accounts, one comes away with an appreciation of these people as individuals, folks not to be regarded as victims but as people meeting the challenges of life just like everyone else. The overarching theme of *Living with Stuttering: Stories, Basics, Resources, and Hope* is that there is always hope for people who stutter.

Who would be interested in these stories? People who stutter; their families, friends, and acquaintances; and anyone who is interested in the human condition will find them fascinating. *Living with Stuttering: Stories, Basics, Resources, and Hope* is most appropriate as a supplemental text for college courses in: introduction to communication disorders (or speech-language pathology), stuttering or fluency disorders, special education, cultural diversity, living with disabilities or handicaps, or personal narrative. A short appendix in the book offers a view of these stories' value from a college student's perspective.

Not only does *Living with Stuttering: Stories, Basics, Resources, and Hope* provide fascinating verbal snapshots of what it can be like to stutter, but it is a carefully crafted self-help and clinical resource as well. It strives to be authoritative yet readable. *Chapter 1: Introduction* identifies key underpinnings for telling one's personal stories from the newly named area of "narrative psychology." *Chapter 3: Stuttering 101: Some Basics,* written in plain English to the person who stutters, summarizes a great deal of what is currently known about the nature and treatment of stuttering. For individuals who stutter or those who know someone who stutters, various appendices describe where to find more information, how to take stock of one's stuttering, and how and where to get help. For example, one appendix provides a suggested reading/video list for different groups (i.e., adults who stutter, the general public, or speech-language pathologists) who wish to learn more about this condition, and allows them to choose whether to spend ten minutes or several days, weeks, or months on the subject.

Two complementary appendices provide guidelines on how those who stutter can "take stock" of their stuttering as a self-study exercise by telling their own stories and by filling out a short inventory on life perspectives and stuttering. Stuttering self-help or support group members, speech-language pathologists, and others may find these Taking Stock materials especially helpful to self-management or speech therapy.

Contents

Chapter 1: Introduction
Kenneth O. St. Louis
Telling your story has value.   17
Listen to the experts!   22
What do they tell us?   23
A final thought.   25

Chapter 2: Our Stories
Working Now for a New Attitude   31
    Tiffany D. Summerlin
Be Yourself   36
    Kenneth L. Hacker
Onset of Stuttering Late in Life Puzzles Me   40
    Ann Jaffe
Therapies Are Flawed, But Forgiveness Isn't   42
    Gregory John Snyder
That Is Just Me   46
    Matthew W. Wilson
Dreaming Big and Having Fun   49
    Brent Forrest Sturm
I Know All the Theories of Stuttering   54
    Fred A. Lewis
My Speech Difficulty Led Me to Special Children   58
    Verna Jane Corley
My Wife Made the Difference   62
    Michael Keith Baker
"Think Positive"   66
    Paul Douglas Gray

70 The Red Rabbit Ran 'Round the Room
Robert W. Quesal

74 I Thought I Was the Only One
Alta F. Sliger

78 I Didn't Want to Be Different
Michael Sugarman

82 And the Winner Is…
Larry R. Padgett

89 "I Decided Then and There to Become a Speech Therapist…"
Kenneth O. St. Louis

95 The Journey from a Coal Town
Sidney Donald Lee

100 The Gift My Stuttering Gave to Me
Meg Coleman Carpenter

104 I Chose to Swim
Joseph (Jay) L. Hanna

107 A Day in the Life of a Stutterer: Trauma in the Drive-Thru
Jennifer Lee Davis

111 Secrets within Us
Patrick T. Niner

117 No More Constant Dread
Lynn F. Caseman

120 Graduate Orals Proved to Be My Testing Ground
Beth Alyson Costine

124 Practice Makes Perfect
Frank Harrison, Jr.

128 With God All Things Are Possible
Henry Brooks Pratt

132 My Struggles with a "Demon"
Jackson B. (JB) Thomas

Chapter 3: Stuttering 101: Some Basics
Kenneth O. St. Louis

What is stuttering?   139
Who stutters and when?   140
What happens during and because of stuttering?   146
Why do people stutter and how are they different from   148
    people who don't stutter?
How do people cope with or manage their stuttering?   155
How can stutterers be more successful?   173

Appendices

A: References   179
B: Reading and video list: How much do you want   184
    to know? (Kenneth O. St. Louis)
    For adults who stutter
    For the general public and new students of SLP
    For trained speech-language pathologists
C: How and where you can get help for your stuttering   194
    (Kenneth O. St. Louis)
    Taking stock
    Locating resources
D: Bill of Rights and Responsibilities for People who   205
    Stutter
E: Some Thoughts from a Speech-Language Pathology   207
    Student (Crystal D. Hightower)
F: Terminology Pertaining to Fluency and Fluency   211
    Disorders: Guidelines (American Speech-Language
    Hearing Association)

(continued)

219   G: Taking Stock: Telling Your Story of Stuttering
           (Kenneth O. St. Louis)
           Why tell your story?
           How can you tell your story?
           Ready? Get started!
           If you are puzzled about where to start, read on.
           Start your story now if you want.
           Telling Your Story Worksheet

231   H: Taking Stock: Assessing Your Life Perspectives and Stuttering
           (Kenneth O. St. Louis)
           Taking and scoring the SL♦ILP-S
           Some forms and a hypothetical example
           Some pilot data on the SL♦ILP-S

249   **Name Index**

251   **Topic Index**

CHAPTER 1

Introduction

Telling your story has value.

Five years ago, I began a project involving stories of stutterers.* Students in my classes have been conducting spontaneous interviews of people who stutter—or used to stutter—to get their honest, unvarnished, personal stories of stuttering. You might wonder, "Why be concerned about individual stories of stuttering?" After all, if you have talked to a number of people who stutter, you would no doubt be impressed that no two stutterers repeat, prolong, or struggle with their words in exactly the same way. Furthermore, there are thousands of research studies on the topic of stuttering that could probably tell us more precisely about this mysterious condition than a few stories from individuals. My response is very simple. Stuttering is often a critical part of experiencing life for people with this condition. In order to fully understand oneself as a stutterer or someone else who stutters, the stories of stuttering must be *told* and must be *heard*.

> "We enter into stories, we are entered into stories by others, and we live our lives through stories."
>
> —*Michael White*

A new and growing area known as "narrative psychology" explores the ways in which individuals make sense of their world through the stories they live and tell. The way that we make sense out of the experiences we have gives our lives meaning. Jean Mandler introduced the term "nuclear episodes" for those positive or negative experiences that mark turning points in our lives. The remembering and telling of stories about these events does a remarkable thing: it captures for us the precise essence of a host of complex experiences and emotions. For example, suppose a good friend asked you what high school was like for you. You might give an oversimplified explanation including a comment that it's impossible to summarize such a huge group of significant experiences into one neat statement. But, suppose your friend

---

* Please see the Reader's Notes at the end of this chapter for a short discussion on terminology in this book (e.g., "stutterers" versus "people who stutter" and "him/her") and on references.

persisted, "What was high school like?" He really wanted to know what high school meant to your life. Since it is impossible to tell him *all* the exhilarating, run-of-the-mill, or agonizing experiences, chances are you would eventually relate *some* actual experiences (part of your "story") about high school. According to narrative psychology, you would pick stories that would portray your strongest impressions of high school (maybe your first real love, maybe your experience in sports, maybe a course you found unusually interesting or boring). If you hated high school, it would be unlikely that you would include in your story a description of how much fun the pep rallies were. If you especially remembered a teacher who really turned you on to learning, you would probably say something about that teacher and something you did together that helped you reach that impression. In other words, you would talk about some of your "nuclear episodes" from high school.

In addition to allowing us to summarize complex experiences, stories give meaning to what we have done or experienced. Sometimes those meanings are uplifting, such as when we recognize that we have contributed to a higher purpose, when our stories have rich interpretations, or simply when they tell us that life makes sense. It could be argued that people who celebrate or seek out their roots through family reunions, genealogy, or a search for their biological parents are attempting to interweave their own stories into the existing and emerging ones of their extended families. As society becomes more and more fragmented, people are increasingly drawn to preserving their stories for future generations—in the form of autobiographies, memoirs, or collections of personal narratives. Some individuals utilize the services of personal historians who interview them and "ghost write." Trained oral historians also seek out individuals whose experiences they consider valuable and carefully record and archive their stories.

Want more information?

A number of excellent book-length autobiographical accounts of stuttering have been published. One by Fred Murray (first published in 1980) and another by Marty Jezer provide first-person glimpses into these two stutterers' struggles with various types of therapy. Marty Jezer's book, especially, discusses pros and cons of various approaches.

Murray, F. P. (1991). *A Stutterer's Story*. Memphis, TN: Stuttering Foundation of America.

Jezer, M. (1997). *Stuttering: A Life Bound up in Words*. New York: BasicBooks.

John Ahlbach and Vicki Benson also published a collection of seventy-two short narratives in book form through the National Stuttering Project (now the National Stuttering Association). Each of the authors represented had been featured in the NSP newsletter, *Letting Go*.

Ahlbach, J. & Benson, V. (1994). *To Say What is Ours*. Anaheim Hills, CA: National Stuttering Project.

Let me digress for a moment and mention one of my own experiences with stories. As you can see from my story in this book, I grew up in rural northwest Colorado. As a child, my extended family lived in a rural, cattle and sheep ranching community. "Us kids" grew up together, and we shared some amazing experiences together, such as attending a one-room school and getting up at 4:00 am one day each summer to drive our fathers' and uncles' cattle to the National Forest pastures. Many of us have since moved far away and made our lives doing other things. But when we get together, we tell stories and tall tales by the hours from our shared youth. At a reunion a few years ago, we told those stories on video-tape so they would not be lost. This was an incredible experience. The St. Louis family has been very fortunate to discover that through the shared telling, retelling, and hearing of our stories, we can reconnect with one another.

> "If we possess our why of life we can put up with almost any how."
>
> —*Friedrich Nietzsche*

Sometimes our stories are not uplifting, as when there seems to be no unifying purpose in the story parts, when the interpretations are impoverished, or when there seems to be no reason for our experiences. However, telling such stories can be healing. Victor Frankl, a Nazi Holocaust survivor and psychiatrist, said that even the terrible suffering he endured in the concentration camp made sense when conceptualized as a "sacrifice" for some higher purpose. Frankl later developed an approach to treating his patients called "logotherapy" or "meaning therapy."

In the past decade, a group of approaches to counseling, called narrative therapies, has emerged. Using existing and new techniques, they seek in various ways to assist people to change their stories, much as Frankl suggested. People are invited to become "authors" of their own stories, both in metaphorical ways and as actual writers or narrators, and to rewrite them to better include what they need and want. One approach includes "story re-visions," or seeing in a fresh or new way what one's story might consist of. The common thread that runs through many of these approaches is that every person with a problem has a story that is absolutely unique. It is therefore unwise for the therapist to presume to completely understand the person's problem and offer advice before participating in the telling of that story. With the counselor's questions and guidance, the client tells and revises the story, sometimes in a way that neither of them could have anticipated or imagined.

Want more information?

Gerald Monk, John Winslade, Kathie Crocket, and David Epston edited a book by numerous authors and experts in narrative therapy. The book begins with an explanation of narrative therapy and how it works. Stuttering is not mentioned, but there are chapters on using the approach with a number of different disorders and groups.

Monk, G., Winslade, J., Crocket, K. & Epston, D. (Eds.). (1997). *Narrative Therapy in Practice: The Archaeology of Hope*. San Francisco: Jossey-Bass Publishers.

Another useful resource is a book by Allan Parry and Robert Doan. It describes the "Postmodern" approaches, including narrative therapy. The book describes the process of "Re-vision," or changing one's story within a therapeutic environment.

Parry, A. & Doan, R. E. (1994). *Story Re-visions: Narrative Therapy in the Postmodern World*. New York: The Guilford Press.

> "We went from the idea of thinking of people as having problems to the idea of problems having people." —*Michael White and David Epston*

These principles also apply to stories of stuttering and can be the basis for renewed hope and significant gains in the future. Those of us who do or have stuttered can remember significant events that shaped our thoughts, feelings, and reactions to our stuttering. I have only met one person in my life who said he rather enjoyed his stuttering. This fellow's stuttering was not very severe, but he had a repetitive stutter that always amused him— "cracked him up," he said. By contrast, virtually all of the rest of us are not pleased with the fact that we stuttered, but we learned to live and cope with it. If we were all to tell our stories, some of us would tell of challenges that we faced and how we learned to speak with a feeling of pride and accomplishment. Yet others will remember speech and social events that terrified or overwhelmed us and think of the times when we truly suffered. Our stories are determined by the totality of our experiences with stuttering.

Importantly, our stories are never finished. Next year, or ten years hence, our stories will be different. Several years ago, Robert Gooden, a stutterer and member of the National Stuttering Project, a support group for people who stutter now known as the National Stuttering Association, was quoted on a birthday card sent to me by the organization. It read, "When people ask me if I have stuttered all my life, I always tell them, 'Not yet.'" I taped that card on my office door, and it is still there. As long as we are alive, we have new experiences that can change us and change our stories. Isn't that marvelous? We can change—indeed, we can make progress toward recovery from our stuttering—up to our last breath.

Returning to the interview project, as soon as I read the first few interviews that my students collected, I knew that there was something very powerful and important in these stories. I was touched by the stutterers' honesty, their suffering, their commitment to improvement, their courage, and their successes. The stories inspired and taught me, as a mostly recovered stutterer myself, but also as a speech-language pathologist who has devoted his entire career to better understanding and treating stuttering. There were also stories of hopelessness, pessimism, and pain, the kind of experiences we don't usually read about in most textbooks on fluency disorders. As I noted at the beginning of this chapter, I have been analyzing interviews now for five years. We have analyzed the major themes expressed, the words used, and the content of the ideas expressed. The results of these efforts are fascinating, but they don't capture the power of the stories. To appreciate the richness of the interviews, you have to read them. That is precisely why I decided to compile these stories and write this book. I wanted everyone to hear the real stories that stutterers have to tell.

> "...Each person's story becomes self legitimizing ...When one person tries to silence the legitimate voice of another, this is done invariably by throwing into question that person's only resource for discerning reality, his/her own judgment. All those who are thrown into that position of self-doubt are being thrown out of their own stories and robbed of their own voices." —*Alan Parry and Robert Doan*

I asked my students to reflect on what they had learned by writing about their experiences arranging, tape-recording, and writing verbatim transcripts of the interviews. This experience often touched them in ways that none of my lectures nor their previous reading and observing had done. The students' reactions varied, of course, but most agreed that sitting down and talking to someone (even over the telephone) made the problem of stuttering truly real for them, often for the first time. The Story Editor, Crystal Hightower, who read all the interviews, carried out content analyses on most of them, and then helped mold the oral interviews into first-person stories for this book, summarized the experience and its impact on her as an undergraduate speech-language pathology student in *Appendix E: Some Thoughts from a Speech-Language Pathology Student.*

Listen to the experts!

After deciding to write and prepare this book, I contacted stutterers who had told the students fascinating, uplifting, and hopeful stories and asked them if they would like to share their stories with the world. Nearly everyone I contacted was delighted to do so.

What follows are the stories of twenty-five adults who know very well what stuttering is and what it feels like. As I mentioned, these stories are not representative of all of the people you might meet who stutter. Some of the people I did not contact have stories that are sad and discouraging, stories of lifelong struggle, suffering, and ridicule. I do not want the reader of this book to assume that such stories do not exist—they do. But so do stuttering stories of courage, hope, and encouragement. This book features the latter. Though these people may have suffered, they made great strides in overcoming the handicaps that afflicted them.

As you read their accounts, you will no doubt be impressed that some have very few, if any, vestiges of earlier complications from stuttering. You may also conclude that some of the individuals still have a way to go in order to completely manage or overcome their problems. It will become clear that there is not one apparent way to overcome the problem. Some, like me, required speech therapy. Others had the wisdom and insight to manage their problems alone or with the help of family, teachers, colleagues, or friends. Speech-language pathologists who read the accounts will undoubtedly identify "remedies" which they could easily and authoritatively conclude were not the ideal recoveries. Still, we must remember that throughout all but the last fraction of history, there was no professional treatment for stuttering, and that is still true for the majority of the world's population today. Courageous people have been overcoming stuttering since the beginning of time, and they continue today.

What do they tell us?

At the beginning of the next chapter, *Tiffany Summerlin* narrates some of her difficult experiences and emotions as a person who rarely stutters openly as well as her progress in coming to grips with it. *Kenneth Hacker* tells tales of his life as a stutterer in rural West Virginia and how he has learned to live a productive life in spite of it. *Ann Jaffe's* unique stuttering problem began during her 90s, opening the possibility of a neurogenic component, but such is not evident in her story. *Greg Snyder* relates how some early painful memories have made him a more forgiving person. He also offers a unique commentary on speech therapy from the perspective of a stutterer who is also a speech-language pathologist. *Matt Wilson* speaks from the perspective of a college football player whose early fear of stuttering gave way to accep-

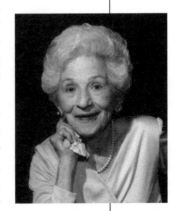

Ann Jaffe.

tance. *Brent Sturm* also learned on his own how to manage a stuttering problem that he says began after a head injury during kindergarten and reflects a psychological problem.

Fred Lewis provides powerful and personal insights into a number of different speech therapy approaches and explains why a nonavoidance approach worked best for him. *Verna Corley* became aware of her stuttering (and/or cluttering) through daily interaction with children as a special education teacher. *Mike Baker* reveals some of the trauma of growing up with a stutter where there was confusion about it in the family, and how the unconditional acceptance and support of his wife made a tremendous difference. *Doug Gray* highlights the therapeutic value of positive thinking by describing his transformation from a withdrawn child to a community leader. *Bob Quesal* reminds us that one must be ready for therapy in order for it to be effective, and shares some insights he has gained as a clinician and a professor of speech-language pathology.

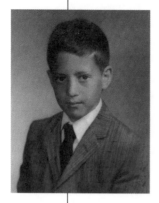

Michael Sugarman.

Alta Sliger's story reveals that stuttering, while troubling day-to-day and difficult to change long term, does not need to prevent us from doing what we choose and enjoy. *Michael Sugarman* relates his journey from a "slow" class in elementary school to founder of the largest self-help and support group for those who stutter. *Larry Padgett* writes of the battle between his stuttering and nonstuttering self as a child and young adult. He goes on to explain how not avoiding stuttering helped him. *Kenneth St. Louis* (me!) describes how he mostly overcame his stuttering (except while speaking a second language) and decided to become a speech-language pathologist as a result of a hard-nosed approach to therapy during his high school and college years. *Sidney Lee* shares how he overcame his problem enough to become an accomplished public speaker. *Meg Coleman Carpenter* tells her story of overcoming stuttering through therapy and accepting the problem as a gift.

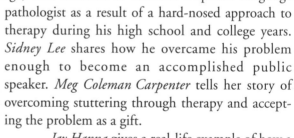
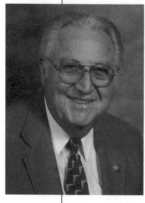

Henry Pratt.

Jay Hanna gives a real-life example of how a "sink or swim" sense of determination helped him overcome and see humor in his stuttering. *Jennifer Davis* provides a glimpse into some of the ongoing struggles and reliefs that a stutterer experiences in daily life. Those who have never stuttered can learn a great deal from her story. *Pat Niner* writes of his doubts about attending his first self-help group for stuttering, which was instrumental in motivating him to help start one himself. *Lynn Caseman,* who felt he was cursed by God as a child, relates a fascinating story of beginning to overcome his stuttering after watching the trembling hands of an eloquent politician. *Beth Costine* tells how her determination to do what she wanted to do, along with speech therapy, was responsible for her success in speaking well in spite of a lifelong stutter. *Frank Harrison* talks of his life as a basketball player and coach, and like several others, identifies ways that he has overcome his stuttering through giving speeches and other strategies. *Henry Pratt* attributes his stuttering to feelings of rejection and describes the uplifting process of becoming a successful pastor and television minister. Finally, *JB Thomas* talks of treating his stuttering "demon" over the years by memorizing speeches and finally realizing that he did not need to speak perfectly.

Numerous themes appear throughout the stories. In addition to some of those I just mentioned, there are stories of pain, humor, rejection, faith, and sympathy. Many different approaches to management of the stuttering are described, some from speech therapy, such as stuttering modification, fluency shaping, and nonavoidance, and some of the individual's or others' own invention, such as talking to trees or being smacked across the back of the hands. One of the most common positive themes is the stutterer's acceptance of stuttering as a part of oneself. It seems when acceptance occurs, strides are made in either changing the stuttering itself or lessening its negative impact on an individual's life.

> **"I never tire of speaking about stuttering. It has been the most intimate experience of my life, and in the lives of almost everyone I have come to know and love in the stuttering community. And what do I love most of all? Telling our stories, of course."**
> *—John Ahlbach*

A final thought.

Tristine Rainer wrote a book called *Your Life as Story.* In it she makes the case that your story is valuable whether you are rich or poor, young or old, famous or ordinary. If you tell your story—your real story—you will discover that, like a novel, it has a beginning, a middle, and an end. The beginning describes who you are, the values that shaped you, and what you wanted. The middle describes the adversaries you encountered as you sought what you wanted. The end describes what you learned from significant turning points in your life. The Rolling Stones say it well, "You can't always get what you want, but if you try some time, you just might find, you get what you need."

Reader's Notes

Terminology

I have chosen to write this book using the designation "stutterer" and "person who stutters" interchangeably. In 1999, I published an article entitled "Person-First Labeling and Stuttering" in the *Journal of Fluency Disorders* that dealt with the issues involved in using either the direct label ("stutterer") versus the person-first label ("person who stutters"). In a nutshell, some advocate person-first terms because they imply that there is much more to a person than the fact that he or she might stutter. I am well aware of the controversy involved in this issue but have made my choice for the following reasons. First and most important, the large amount of data I gathered and reported clearly shows that there is no pejorative or stigmatizing connotation of the term "stutterer" versus "person who stutters" for all but a very small fraction of the population. For the average person, even speech and hearing disordered clients or their parents, there is no difference between the two. In fact, there were a few instances in which respondents slightly favored the term "stutterer." And with some other names, a direct label is preferred, e.g., "composer" over "person who composes." Second, I have never met anyone, and especially no one who works or interacts with those who stutter in a helpful way, who ever used the term "stutterer" in a pejorative way. It simply describes a phenomenon. Third, I believe that the common abbreviations that have appeared, such as "PWS" for "person who stutters," "CWS" for "child who stutters," or "PCWS" for "parent of a child who stutters," are confusing and perhaps have themselves become dehumanizing. Although I stutter, and although I am sensitive to—and do not in any way condone—derogatory and discriminative comments and actions toward anybody who stutters, I would never refer to myself or prefer to be referred to as a "PWS." Fourth, the long person-first versions often make writing awkward, and the abbreviations make possessives, e.g., PWS's or PWSs', difficult to understand.

Also, before you go any further, I would like to say a few words about "gender language." After wrestling with the issue of inclusive language versus ease of reading, I have made the decision to be inconsistent. Sometimes I use "him or her." However, you may encounter sentences that would be awkward if I used that type of "inclusive language." An example would be, "The first thing to remember when interviewing him or her is to make sure that he or she is comfortable and that you are sensitive to his or her needs." Wanting the text to flow smoothly, I decided to use only one pronoun (e.g., "him," *or* "her") in such situations.

References

Appendix A: References lists references used in this book. The reader will note that, except for the "Want more information?" sections, citations or footnotes were generally not provided in the text. I wrote it this way to make it easier to read. Obviously some of the material in this book is original, but part of *Chapter 1: Introduction* and a great deal of *Chapter 3: Stuttering 101: Some Basics* summarize research and thinking of others. All of those individuals are listed in *Appendix A: References*.

CHAPTER 2
Our Stories

Working Now for a New Attitude

I'M NOT AN EXTREME STUTTERER, BUT IT IS ENOUGH TO change and inconvenience my life. To me, stuttering is a very shameful thing. I know that I shouldn't feel that way, but I don't want anybody to know. Outwardly, my speech is pretty smooth, and I work very hard to substitute words I can say for words I can't say easily.

I am too prideful about it. Stuttering has a stigma about it that people who stutter must have something wrong with them. I have always felt like it was shameful to my father. So, that was

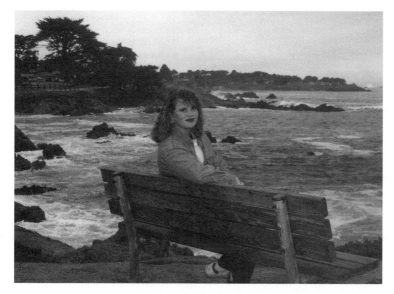

Tiffany relaxes on the Monterey, California, beach.

kind of hard. As a very little girl, I didn't talk much around him because I was afraid of stuttering.

There are so many times and so many situations when I feel like I could help or be welcoming to people, but I don't because of my stuttering. For example, I could say, "Hey, do you want to come to my church?" or "My name is...," but I would just freeze up. I just wouldn't be able to say anything. That is so hard to deal with because I end up feeling really guilty, very worthless. I am very hard on myself that way.

I don't really avoid situations, but I avoid saying things that I really want to say. I end up feeling like I'm missing out on many opportunities. I feel like I fail by not saying things to people. I really feel that it's an important thing to reach out and to be of service to others, but I often fail to do it because I'm so self-conscious. It's not worth the embarrassment or risk of embarrassment.

There have been many life decisions that I have made because I am afraid of the way other people view stutterers. Most people think that there is something wrong with stutterers or that they are less intelligent. I have been known as a very intelligent person and don't feel like I'm stupid. But knowing what other people might think of me makes me feel very insecure about my stuttering.

I was afraid to go to college. I just hated the classroom atmosphere. For example, if anyone asked me to read aloud, I had to "psych" myself up to do it. Usually, I did fine, but sometimes I wished that I could just crawl into a hole and die. I also had to trick myself into maybe going to college; therefore, I participated in a college scholarship pageant. If I won the scholarship, I would be forced to go to college. I didn't end up winning the scholarship, and I just didn't really want to go to college, so I joined the military. I thought that would be the

> **I don't want anybody to know. Outwardly, my speech is pretty smooth, and I work very hard to substitute words I can say for words I can't say easily.**

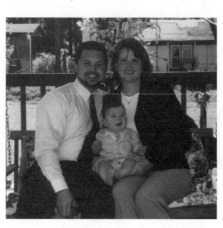

Tiffany with husband Jamie, and baby Nicholas makes three.

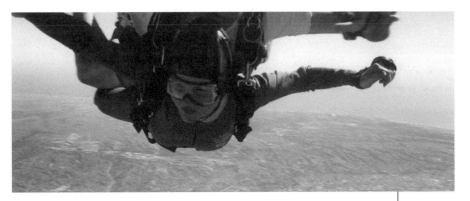

Tiffany skydiving in 1998 near San Diego, California.

easiest thing for me to do to get out of a really small town. Plus, I was drawn to the military environment.

Joining the military proved to be a really good thing for me. Because I do better in high-pressure rather than relaxed and casual atmospheres, I joined the toughest branch, the Marine Corps. I did fine. I was always forced to talk, and required to do it on command. I could do that with ease because I didn't have to choose things to say. I also had to be confident, which helped a little. I did very well in the Marine Corps and within three and a half years I was promoted to E5, which usually took five or six years.

While in the military, I think I tried to throw myself into situations that made me deal with my stuttering. Kind of conquer it. I thought, "I just have to get over this." I signed up for a speech class. We did a few little speeches "impromptu" or we read things aloud. But, for some reason I got scared and said to myself, "I can't take this class anymore!" Sometimes I feel fine getting up in front of people and talking, but other times I just can't do it.

I was afraid to go to college. I just hated the classroom atmosphere. For example, if anyone asked me to read aloud, I had to "psych" myself up to do it. Usually, I did fine, but sometimes I wished that I could just crawl into a hole and die.

After leaving the military, I also pushed myself into jobs that put me in situations where I would have to deal with my stuttering. For example, my first job was as a sales person at Victoria's Secret. There were times when it was hard for me to ask customers certain questions. If I had to say, "Would you like to apply for a Victoria's Secret credit card?" I couldn't do it sometimes, so I just wouldn't say it regardless of the repercussions. Also there are many times when "my vocabulary fails me." (Too chicken to try the word

I know, I act the ignorant party.) I feel like I'm shortchanging myself because I know these things, but I'm too embarrassed to try and risk being ashamed.

My fear about stuttering also often changes people's perceptions of me. They often seem to think that I'm quiet because I think I'm better than they are, but that is not it at all. I would just love to talk to people, but sometimes it's so hard. Through the years I think people just kind of left me alone. I didn't really have many friends and didn't really develop my social skills like I should have because I was so terrified.

> I would just love to talk to people, but sometimes it's so hard. Through the years I think people just kind of left me alone. I didn't really have many friends and didn't really develop my social skills like I should have because I was so terrified.

Now, most of the friends that I have know that I stutter, and it is so much easier. My husband never knew until I told him six months into our marriage. These days, if I stumble over a word, he'll encourage me, "Come on, you can do it." That helps me so much. There have been so many different times that I wanted to tell people because I felt it would help me. If people know, I usually don't have a problem. If I meet someone who knows that I stutter, I probably wouldn't stutter because I wouldn't feel like I had to perform in front of him or her. But, it would be kind of awkward to meet somebody and say, "Hey, I stutter, my name is…" To me that would be so hard.

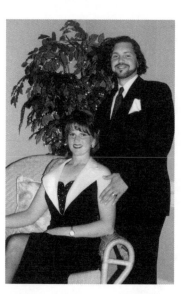

Tiffany and Jamie.

Like many who stutter, I have also been in search of the "magical cure." I remember one time when I thought that I had discovered it. I thought that I wouldn't stutter anymore if I took a really deep breath before I started talking. I guess it worked a few times for me, but I soon discovered it wasn't that helpful.

Now, I am working to get to the point when I can just make light of it and joke about my stuttering. However, it is sometimes still very serious for me. I know other people who have stuttered and just say, "Huh, oh well," and go on with life. They say "whatever it takes," even if it means people looking at them funny.

I admire that in people and wish that I could do that. That is now what I am working towards, but I think that that attitude is easier for some personalities than others. Another thing I wish for is that people would treat me as a person, not a stutterer. I am a person, a woman, a wife, a mother, a veteran, and more. Stuttering is just a part.

Author: Tiffany D. Summerlin.

Tiffany is a twenty-six-year-old stay-at-home mother of one son and she enjoys photography. Originally from Myrtle Point, Oregon, she now resides in Morgantown, West Virginia. Tiffany spent five years in active duty with the US Marine Corps. She and her husband, also a former Marine, met while on active duty in Iwakuni, Japan.

401-001-TR-ST-001-2001

Be Yourself

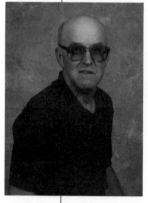

Ken, much as he looks today, at home and at the senior center.

I AM NOW A SIXTY-EIGHT-YEAR-OLD RETIRED LUMBER STACKER AND consider myself to be a moderate-to-severe stutterer. I spent most of my childhood on the Greenbrier River, back on Bening's Knob and up Liquor Bottoms. Back in those days there wasn't speech therapy. In fact, I went to my first school in Fenwick when I was seven. My dad lived back in the woods when I was younger, and it was too far to walk. So, when we moved to Fenwick, we started in school down there.

The first time I had the chance for speech therapy was in the military. They thought that they might send me to speech school, but they changed their mind. I just had six months to go, and I wasn't going to stay in the military, so from their standpoint there wasn't any need to send me, I guess.

I still to this day have problems saying my own name. I'll tell you, my name is one of the hardest things I ever have to say. Yes, sir. I can say the complete names of my friends Bob or Stanley or Gene or Frank, but my own name, it sticks. I don't know why, but it has always been that way.

A few other things are hard for me to say. I know when something is coming that I can't say. I can go down to Dairy Queen or McDonald's or Shoney's and try to order something. If it is something I can't say, I'll just spell it out. I just laugh like I said it, and it doesn't bother me. Sometimes I'll say "c-o-f-f-e-e" and they will say, "Come again?" and I'll just spell it again. "Tomato" does me the same way. If I want to order it on a sandwich, I'll spell it. They'll say, "What'd you say?" and I'll say, "t-o-m-a-t-o." It doesn't bother me; I just go ahead and spell it anywhere I go.

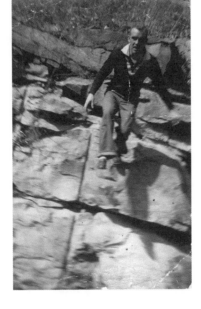

Ken in 1965 at age thirty-five. Both then and now, Ken likes to keep physically active.

I was always a good speller in school. Oh heck, back in my day I used to be a pretty good speller. We would have spelling contests and the winner in those days would get fifteen or twenty-five cents. And buddy, I made sure I got it. So, if I can't say it, I spell it.

A lot of people think that just because I can't talk, I'm not intelligent. But I am as smart as the rest of them. If anybody wants to know anything about the Good Book, I can tell 'em. I don't know why God gave me a good mind for that, but I can now quote over eight hundred scriptures easy.

I can read out loud to myself easy, but reading out loud to other people is tough. I don't know why. I can sit here and read out loud to myself easy because the words just come and my mind can't wander. To read out loud in a group is different, the words just stick in my head. I never did understand that. Another thing I don't understand is with singing. I can't sing much, but it seems like you can go right ahead and, I don't care where you are, you don't stutter when you're singing.

I can say the complete names of my friends Bob or Stanley or Gene or Frank, but my own name, it sticks. I don't know why, but it has always been that way.

I've stood up in church at one of those deacon or ordination things in front of a hundred people. I do a lot of stuff like that. I have to stand up and give my name. Everybody just sits and waits; I can't spell my name for them. I'll eventually say it, "Kenneth Hacker," which is really hard. I'm not scared or anything, I just get tense. I'll sometimes even stutter through the prayer. If

I can't say a word, I'll just skip it. The Lord knows what I'm trying to say anyway. He knows what I'm talking about.

The people in my life all react differently to my stuttering. My dad would always tell me to shut up. Dad didn't really help me. He was an oddball is what I like to call it. I liked Dad, but back in those days, you didn't have a close relationship with your dad. My mom didn't say anything much about my stuttering either. She was very understanding. There are some people who I know real well and when I start to say something, they will say it for me. It doesn't bother me, it tickles me; I just laugh. My wife would jump right in when she thought that I was going to say something, she'd go ahead and say it. I'd just shut up. It wasn't that I couldn't say it; she was just helping me. With other people, I could tell them that I couldn't say something and to hold on, and they would just sit there and not seem to care.

> I'll sometimes even stutter through the prayer. If I can't say a word, I'll just skip it. The Lord knows what I'm trying to say anyway. He knows what I'm talking about.

I was an automatic lumber stacker and ran this big eighty-foot-long machine. They would put the lumber on and we would push the button to straighten it up in the pile. The boys there never said anything. I could out-work most of them on the job to start with, I was as smart as the rest of them, and they didn't really put me down at any time.

I never had any trouble socializing with people either. Growing up, I got more girlfriends than some of the other boys did. I don't know why, I guess that's just the way it was. I just socialize anywhere. I just get right in there. I was in the Baptist Youth Fellowship. We'd go to Baptist Camp, and there would be one hundred and fifty kids there. I must have been forty or forty-five then and none of them could out-swim me or out-run me. They just couldn't believe it. The boys would come up and tell me what a good time they had. I've always been around people I don't know and got along pretty well.

I also go to the senior center every day now. I go just to eat and socialize. There are generally thirty of us, and I talk to everybody, both the men and the women. It's a friendly group. Everybody hollers at me to come over and they don't say a bad word about me.

Most of them can't understand why I still ride my bike there. I ride my bike or walk downtown most of the time if it's pretty. I try to keep fit even now. I got a load of logs just to have something to do, and my gosh, did I ever get something to do! I have most of them sawed up though.

Stuttering has never held me back. I never let it bother me. I just pay real close attention to my speech. I learned real fast to never be intimidated by it.

Author: Kenneth L. Hacker.
Kenneth is a sixty-eight-year-old retiree of Georgia Pacific from Richwood, West Virginia. He has happily enjoyed camping, bicycling, swimming, and scuba diving for eighteen years. He suggests that you be yourself, love the Lord, and maintain good health.

402-001-TR-ST-001-2001

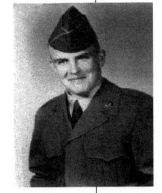

Ken in the US Army.

Onset of Stuttering
Late in Life Puzzles Me

I HAVEN'T THE SLIGHTEST IDEA WHY I STARTED TO STUTTER IN MY nineties. I have no reason for it, and I wasn't upset. To tell you the truth, I was as surprised as anybody else when I started to stutter. At first I attributed it to maybe being overwrought about my physical condition, but then I overruled that because I remembered that I had been in this physical condition for quite a few years, during which time I did not stutter.

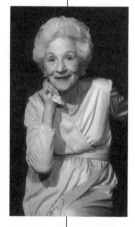

Ann Jaffe has a flair for fun, as this photo of her at a party suggests.

Just suddenly when I got up one morning I started to speak, and I was stuttering. That was about two months ago and there haven't been any new medical conditions that I have noticed. But to be sure, I went to my ophthalmologist, and he said my eyes were good. I also went to my medical doctor, and he said my pressure was good, my temperature was fine, and my heart and lungs were good. I do get swelling in my feet, for which I take a diuretic. He suggested a blood count because the ophthalmologist said something about maybe I had a stroke. That sort of floored me, and I am waiting for the report now of the blood test he took. But I am fine other than that. I really am.

I try not to stutter. When I speak to people on the phone or am with them personally, I try not to stutter, and check with them by asking them if they can understand me. They say that I am speaking very nicely, and they encourage me. So I feel I am making some progress. I know that when I am home alone, I will speak louder, as though there were somebody here with me. I speak much better than I am doing now. I don't know if I am self-conscious about it or if that is part of the stuttering. So I check with friends by asking them how I sound when I am talking with them. That helps.

There is no history of stuttering in my family. No one as far as I go back. Nobody ever stuttered or had any other types of speech problems or language problems. It is not a hereditary thing, I am positive of that. I think if I continue to think about it, I am going to beat this. I am very optimistic about it.

Even if the stuttering does not decrease, I would not consider getting treatment because I am not worried about it at all. I am more worried when I misplace something.

If I make an effort not to speak quickly, I speak better. Because my hearing is not 100 percent, people sometimes get irritated, and that could make me begin to stutter. I become frustrated. I don't think I have a major problem other than that. A slower pace definitely helps me.

More than my speech, I have anxiety about my family members who are ill, and that's a real anxiety. I thank God that I don't have any financial problems and that I don't have to look to anybody to help me pay my rent or food bills or whatever I need. I just have to ask for explanations about a lot of things I don't understand.

It is not a hereditary thing, I am positive of that. I think if I continue to think about it, I am going to beat this. I am very optimistic about it.

Author: Ann Jaffe.

Ann, or "Granny," as her family calls her, is "somewhere between ninety-five and one-hundred." She thinks it is fun to keep them guessing. This statement reflects Ann's fun-loving attitude. She likes to dance and party, always has a positive outlook, is kind and tells a great story. Although born in Europe, Ann has lived most of her life in Baltimore and the Washington, DC, area where she currently resides.

403-001-TR-ST-001-2001

Therapies Are Flawed, But Forgiveness Isn't

I REALLY CAN'T SAY AS EASILY AS I MIGHT HAVE IN THE PAST HOW stuttering has affected my life. Now, in 1999, I'm thinking more sociologically, and about how stuttering affects an entire population. Furthermore, because I've always been a stutterer, I don't know that I'm able to make comparisons of stuttered versus non-stuttered life experiences. I do think, however, that probably the biggest way that my stuttering has affected me is by giving me a very distinct picture of human nature.

> I think the thing that stuttering has made me is more forgiving; perhaps more than anything else, it has changed me in the area of acceptance and forgiveness. It has empowered me, and given me the strength to forgive those who do not understand.

I think the thing that stuttering has made me is more forgiving; perhaps more than anything else, it has changed me in the area of acceptance and forgiveness. It has empowered me, and given me the strength to forgive those who do not understand. Reactions are certainly very negative toward the person who stutters because they are speaking in a fashion that is perceived as abnormal, as well as all sorts of secondary behaviors that are perceived as funny. When there's an entire population that experiences similar issues based on related prejudicial situations, it seems that a minority population is born—a stuttering population that is yet unrecognized. Just within the past three or four—maybe five—years I guess, I've started to better accept human nature, prejudice, and discrimination that happen.

I remember there was a time when I think I was a sophomore or junior in college. A friend and I went to a McDonald's on a Sunday evening because the school's cafeteria was closed. When I was ordering something, I was stuttering. The server kept on looking at my friend and asking my friend what I was saying. That was the first time that I actually saw, almost in slow motion, what was occurring. It was like a specific act of prejudice—because the server believed I could not talk, or social intolerance—because the server didn't have the extra few seconds to let me speak the only way I can.

That incident was a perceptual breakthrough for me. I can only project, but it seems like the server guy was feeling awkward or something, such that he felt he needed to speak with a similar-speaking, fluent individual to interpret. I was able to recognize that the majority of the time, the fluent listener—or even the stuttering listener—doesn't necessarily have malicious intentions. It's just such a social abnormality that they aren't sure what to do with the communicative event. Even though stuttering very rarely affects the intelligibility, it must be unsettling that the timing and comfort of the exchange are imperfect.

After college, I had another memorable experience. I was in the process of applying to different universities for speech-pathology graduate programs—and one college required an entire day of testing and interviews. I met the entire departmental faculty and took great care—using every technique I could—to speak as fluidly as possible. The lady in charge of the interview process seemed very enthusiastic about my contributions to group discussions, as well as the opinions I shared in personal conversations.

> When I was ordering something, I was stuttering. The server kept on looking at my friend and asking my friend what I was saying. That was the first time that I actually saw, almost in slow motion, what was occurring.

Greg enjoys travel and archeology. Here, he is in Corinth, Greece, exploring some ruins.

I remember speaking to her, and getting stuck with a block that lasted a couple of seconds. I noticed a physical response on her face—and for the rest of the day she essentially ignored me. She no longer sought my opinions or contributions, and didn't even bother to show up for my final personal interview. It seemed as if after seeing my stuttering, she immediately developed a negative opinion of me.

Ironically, the thing that I found most perplexing is that not only was this department chair a woman, but a member of an accepted minority group at that. I would have assumed that she would be more sensitive to issues of prejudice, discrimination, and societal marginalization because of some experiences that she may have had to face in her own life.

Recently, I've just been thinking about how I've never seen a person who stutters live a seemingly happy existence that hasn't learned how to forgive. It's forgiveness of others, but also, of ourselves—as we try to live our lives with our stuttering and our attempts at therapy. I think the offshoot of a lot of therapies is that the stutterers feel guilty because they are not fulfilling their expectations; they feel shame because they aren't able to perform in the fashion that they are told is possible. This is a tremendously negative situation for the stuttering population. One time an advisor at school pointed out that for many therapy approaches, the therapist says that stuttering is essentially a choice—if clients use all of the techniques, they will speak fluently. But, if they aren't speaking fluently, it's the client's fault because they supposedly aren't using those techniques. In my life, I know for certain that from time to time, even if I use the most perfectly crafted therapy technique, I'll still find myself stuttering. Using fluency-enhancing techniques is like trying to cross your fingers on both hands at every syllable; it takes consistent conscious control—and I've yet to sacrifice my psyche to that idol because the payoff is too little.

The whole notion and practice of "therapy" is sometimes troubling to me. The techniques are not sufficiently scientifically proven to be effective. Secondly, the entire stuttering treatment paradigm is pretty much untestable. If it's assumed, and I think it should be, that stuttering is some form of a neurological or central nervous

> **I remember speaking to her, and getting stuck with a block that lasted a couple of seconds. I noticed a physical response on her face—and for the rest of the day she essentially ignored me.**

system dysfunction, forms of therapy that use behavioral techniques are essentially fighting the symptoms and not the problem. So immediately, it seems as if that's a flawed approach. But, if you're the speech therapist, the emphasis on stuttering behaviors is absolutely fabulous. The therapist can stress how, "It's up to you to make sure that you're fluent," and if treatment seems successful, the therapist can feel, "Wow, look at me. I'm a super therapist!" If the therapy is unsuccessful, it's the client's burden: "Well, look at him; you know he wasn't using my targets." So what kind of "therapy" is that?

> It's forgiveness of others, but also, of ourselves—as we try to live our lives with our stuttering and our attempts at therapy.

Author: Gregory John Snyder.
Greg is a twenty-six-year-old doctoral student in Communication Sciences and Disorders and married his wife, Courtney, in 1997. His interests and hobbies are many, and include philosophy and theology, as well as water sports, nature, animals, and auto racing.

404-001-TR-ST-001-2001

That Is Just Me

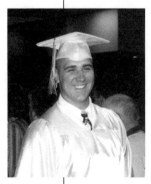

The happy high school graduate in 1996.

EVER SINCE I WAS A LITTLE KID I HAVE ALWAYS STUTTERED, SLURRED my speech, or said "like so" a lot. I always slurred up reading. I also always said my vowels wrong, so it hindered my reading young because I stuttered. In elementary school they put me in a speech class for an hour once a week. I would go into her little room and we would talk. She would ask me about my week and I would just talk to her. The lady in speech class told me that my thoughts were going faster than my talking and that was why I would start to slur my speech. She would tell me, "Slow down, Matt," and to think about what I was going to say first. All that we would do was talk for an hour, or maybe I would read an article out of the paper, just to practice my speech. My stuttering didn't die down much then, but what I learned about slowing down ended up being very important to me.

I don't stutter a lot now. I still stutter but not nearly as bad as I used to. I just talk slower. That is the main thing that you have to tell people is that if they start to stutter, to slow down and think about their speech, then just say it, to talk a little slower. I will still start to stutter if I am really nervous about something that I am saying or if I am telling a really exciting story. I start speaking so fast to get it out or if I am nervous, I am scared not to stutter, so I do.

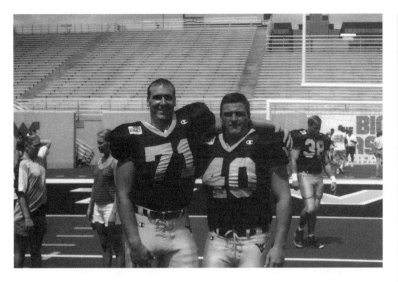

Matt Wilson, on the left, with roommate Wes Ours on Media Day 1998. Both play football for the West Virginia University Mountaineers.

I play football for the West Virginia Mountaineers. If a reporter comes to talk to me and ask me questions, I may have a hard time sitting there and thinking about all of the right answers off the top of my head, and end up stuttering. Although I am trying to say the right words and make a good impression, I still end up stuttering with the camera in front of my face.

My parents also taught me to slow down and think about my speech. They were very supportive, especially my mom. She would read magazines and find people who stuttered and overcame their stuttering, for example, James Earl Jones who played Darth Vader's voice on *Star Wars*. James Earl Jones stuttered really badly as he grew up. In college he slowed down his thought process and started talking more clearly and slower. Now he is a famous voice. My parents supported me by pointing out people like him to me. My mom would read articles like them and send them to me or give them to me. All of the articles would basically tell me to slow down and concentrate.

One Friday night before a game against Syracuse, I called home and talked to my dad. We had talked about the game and their supposedly unblockable defensive end. He said, "How are you going to block him, Matt?" I said, "Well, I guess I will talk at him and try to get in on his focus." My father said, "Well, don't stutter at him or he might laugh at you. Just joking."

> Stuttering has taught me to really be able to pick out who is a true person or a true friend. There are some people who just like to crack on you to make others laugh and be really mean.

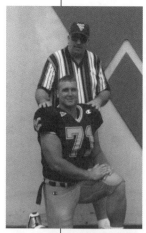

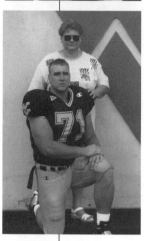

My father can joke around with me like that and it doesn't bother me.

As a little kid, people always picked on me, but these were people who didn't know what stuttering was. Classmates would laugh at me, which was real hard growing up because it made me scared to go up in front of the class or ask a question or talk to a pretty girl. But as I got older, I overcame it. Now, I have a stuttering problem, and that is the way I speak. That is just me. It doesn't really bother me now to stutter in front of people. It bothers me, but not like it did as a little kid.

Stuttering has taught me to really be able to pick out who is a true person or a true friend. There are some people who just like to crack on you to make others laugh and be really mean. Your true friends can crack on you, but you know that they are always around for you and will help you out. All of my friends from home always tell me to slow down when I start to talk fast and stutter, and I start talking slower.

Stuttering made me learn a lot about myself, too. I learned how to cope with people who crack on me and the courage to learn to deal with getting up in front of class and talking. It is hard, but you overcome it and when you are done, it feels a lot better because you talked in front of the class. And sometimes it comes out on the bad end, but then you just learn a lot about yourself and who you are.

Author: Matthew W. Wilson.

Matt is a twenty-three-year-old student at West Virginia University in Morgantown. He received a full athletic scholarship to play football and is pursuing a degree in landscape architecture. From Canton, Ohio, he is the son of Jerry and Sue Wilson and the brother of Tonya. Matt enjoys outdoor life, cooking, relaxing, and playing many sports in addition to football.

405-006-TR-ST-001-2001

Dreaming Big
and Having Fun

First of all I would like to say what I think stuttering is. For me, I honestly think that it is a psychological, mental, confidence problem. I do not think that it is a physiological thing for most people. I believe that it is something that you can control and that the more confident and sure of yourself you are, the easier it will be. Confidence has everything to do with it.

I know that if I think that I am going to stutter on a word, I do; my attitude and mood also affect it. When I have more of a positive attitude or am more confident, I really do not stutter. If I am kind of unsure of myself, I can't get it out.

No other member of my family agrees with me, but I believe that I started to stutter in kindergarten after I had an accident. I cracked my head open when I fell off some bleachers and I had stitches and a neck brace. I had to go to school in a neck brace with half of my head shaved and stitches hanging out. I thought that was when it started, even though I don't think my stuttering is physiologically based.

I know for sure that I stuttered in the fourth grade. I remember difficulties having to lead the Pledge of Allegiance at that time. My teacher picked a different student every day to begin the Pledge. That day she said, "Brent stand up. Do the Pledge." I was like, "Oh, I have to say the Pledge, oh no." I had to start with,

> That day she said, "Brent stand up. Do the Pledge." I was like, "Oh, I have to say the Pledge, oh no." I had to start with, "I pledge allegiance to the flag...," and I knew that I couldn't say "I."

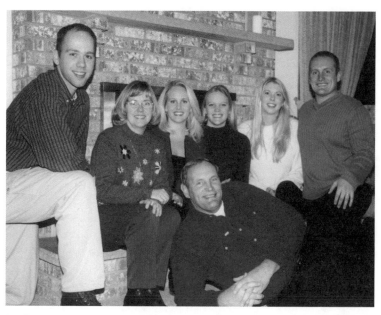

The Sturm family celebrates Christmas 2000 (l-r): brother-in-law Kevin, mom Lora, sister Shelley, sister Kelley, wife Jaime, and author Brent. Dad, Larry, reclines in front.

"I pledge allegiance to the flag...," and I knew that I couldn't say "I." You just have to say "I pledge" and then everyone else chimes in. I tried to start with "pledge" instead of "I" and everyone said, "Why didn't you start with 'I'?"

At this same time I remember starting speech therapy classes. We would talk and that seemed to help a lot. I liked going with my therapist to speech class because we worked on certain words and reading. I loved to read and read aloud to her. I think the sessions helped me a ton. I went up until sixth grade, and I don't remember going very much in middle school until starting up again after a school spelling bee incident.

My class was having a spelling bee, and I stuttered on a word. I knew how to spell it, but I stuttered and my teacher said, "No, that's wrong." I said, "What do you mean that's wrong?" My classmates told her that I just do that and it's not a big deal. She referred me that day to speech therapy and kicked me out of her class. I guess she felt bad that the whole class sided with me and rallied against her.

> I ended up going to her every Friday for a month, and I don't think that it did anything. She would just say, "Here is a list of words, say them all to me. You have all day." Since it was just the two of us sitting at a table saying words, I didn't stutter on any of them.

When I met with the new therapist, she told me that my teacher had said that I had some real bad problems. I told her that I had just stuttered on a word that I was spelling aloud. I ended up going to her every Friday for a month, and I don't think that it did anything. She would just say, "Here is a list of words, say them all to me. You have all day." Since it was just the two of us sitting at a table saying words, I didn't stutter on any of them. I don't think she helped me at all. She wasn't anything like my wonderful fourth-grade therapist. She had a huge impact.

I developed my own tactics for dealing with my stuttering. Now I try not to avoid a word that I know that I may stutter on, but I used to do that. I was smart enough to know other words to use. These days, I try to go ahead and say the word. I feel when I am going to stutter, and I try to calm down and say it. But, I never just say it. I usually go ahead and stutter two or three times and then say it. I know that if I would take a little time to calm down, the pause wouldn't even be noticeable, but I just don't do it.

I hate it when people finish my sentences for me. That is the worst possible thing that you can do. Depending on my mood, sometimes it can make me really mad. For example, someone filling in a word when we're fighting is especially maddening. I know that I can do it, so I'll just say, "Please don't do that."

> I hate it when people finish my sentences for me. That is the worst possible thing that you can do. Depending on my mood, sometimes it can make me really mad. For example, someone filling in a word when we're fighting is especially maddening. I know that I can do it, so I'll just say, "Please don't do that."

I've also developed ways to deal with stuttering in front of people who notice it. It usually takes two or three weeks for them to notice and I'll be like, "Darn, I was trying not do to that." I will just bring it up and talk about it for a minute and they will be like, "Oh, okay."

It kind of waned off in high school. For the past ten or fifteen years I haven't had any major situations. I feel like I can totally control it about eighty-five percent of the time. So, I just stutter every now and then. Maybe on the phone or on some difficult, long word. I may get stuck on the first letter. I am not scared at all about stuttering. For example, I went into the office the other day, and they said four or five people were coming for lunch and to have a presentation ready for after lunch. I only had an hour to prepare, and it wasn't a big deal at all.

I don't get scared to get in front of people. I'm not shy or anything like that, at all, or even a little bit. And talking in front of people, even in large groups of people or one-on-one. No problem. I teach classes at the university, and I've always taught swimming lessons and CPR, lifeguarding, and first aid. I've presented in little groups and I've been in front of big groups of people to talk. The number of people doesn't really make that much of a difference. I don't know if it should or not. I don't go into situations thinking, oh, I'm gonna stutter really bad. That thought never enters my mind. I don't think it's ever made me more shy or hesitant to participate or get involved.

There are certain things that make my stuttering better or worse even today. When I'm real sure of myself and I'm the "big stud," it doesn't happen. My stuttering goes through "comfort stages" with people. When I first meet you, I stutter. Then, I get to know you a little, and I won't. Then, I really get to know you, and I will again. When my girlfriend would break up with me and I'd be all down low, then it would come out more. If I could tell that things weren't going well with a girl that I was seeing, I would stutter more. In my opinion, social and emotional factors are everything.

It doesn't embarrass me now like it used to. Anyhow, people who don't know that I stutter probably just think that I'm doing it because I am excited. I tell myself, they don't know that I stutter and everyone does it when they are excited anyway. Today, I kind of wish that I didn't do it, but it is not a big deal. It is part of what makes me me. I accept that. I don't think that stuttering has made that big a difference in my life. I am a very outgoing person. I don't think that it has stopped me from approaching anyone, male or female. And, I don't think that I have received any special treatment because of it.

Living with stuttering, I have developed an ear

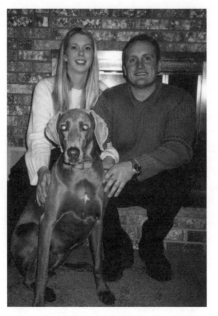

Misty poses with her caretakers Jaime and Brent.

for picking up on other stutterers. When I am talking to another person who stutters, I can kind of feel what he is doing and going through. I'd never finish a sentence for him; I am just calm and listen. I see people on the news and on TV doing the different cues that I learned in therapy and I'm thinking, "Hey, he's doing a cue." I know that is what they are doing, but I don't think the average person even notices. I think stutterers consider these outward behaviors as a lot more important and apparent than other people do. A lot of people just don't care. It doesn't bother them. Everyone stutters a little every now and then anyway.

My stuttering goes through "comfort stages" with people. When I first meet you, I stutter. Then, I get to know you a little and I won't. Then, I really get to know you and I will again.

Author: Brent Forrest Sturm.

Brent is a twenty-seven-year-old Therapy Recreation Specialist and Aquatics Specialist. He is also beginning his own private aquatic therapy practice. Brent takes pride in his strong family bond with his wife, Jaime, his two sisters, and parents. Brent is from Charleston, West Virginia, and enjoys weight training, mountain biking, snowboarding, martial arts, and all other aggressive sports. Brent firmly believes that stuttering is directly related to self-confidence and personal comfort zones.

406-001-TR-ST-001-2001

I Know All
the Theories of Stuttering

I'VE BEEN STUTTERING SINCE AROUND FIVE YEARS OLD, ALTHOUGH I was not aware at the time I was having a speech problem. At about age eight people brought it to my attention. Then I recognized totally that I was speaking kind of funny and not like the other kids.

> **He recovered on his own, without any formal therapy, mainly because he let nothing get in his way, and never avoided speaking situations.**

I had a fairly typical childhood, I suppose, and am the youngest of three sons. I always considered my oldest brother someone who stuttered also. He recovered on his own, without any formal therapy, mainly because he let nothing get in his way, and never avoided speaking situations.

As for me, I began avoiding people and speaking situations of all kinds throughout high school and continuing into college. College was probably the hardest period of my life in terms of stuttering, and I avoided daily almost every challenging speaking situation.

College was also the first time I had any speech therapy at all. I grew up in a small town in the South, and there were no speech therapists there at the time. I was kind of groping for answers to stuttering, and there was a speech clinic in the college I attended that I went to, off and on, for a couple of semesters. I don't think it did too much for me at the time, and I don't even remember the type of approach that they used.

After college I worked for a couple of years in a hospital and then went to graduate school. I had a smattering of therapy in graduate school, consisting of some relaxation-based therapy and a one-week intensive course up in New York based on a passive airflow approach. Looking back on it now, in my opinion anyway, both were absolutely the wrong approaches to the problem of stuttering. At any rate, they didn't do much for me, and may in fact have delayed my seeking more appropriate therapy.

I got married at age twenty-five, while still in graduate school. About eight years ago I went back to therapy involving a combined approach of fluency shaping, some stuttering modification, and breathing exercises. Although I saw some progress, it wasn't until about four years ago, when I started working with a therapist who trained under Joseph Sheehan at the University of California, Los Angeles (UCLA), that I started to make substantial progress on the road to recovery. Sheehan developed an avoidance reduction approach, which basically incorporates many of the elements of Van Riper's stuttering modification approach.

The avoidance reduction approach is to come totally out of the closet, as it were, about stuttering, trying not to hide anything about our speech. Basically, most of our abnormal speech patterns are just remnants of tricks that we've learned over the years to avoid the moment of stuttering. Of course, all of our tricks and all of our patterns are not common. For a lot of people who stutter, one pattern may be shared, such as a loss of eye contact,

> Looking back on it now, in my opinion anyway, both were absolutely the wrong approaches to the problem of stuttering. At any rate, they didn't do much for me, and may in fact have delayed my seeking more appropriate therapy.

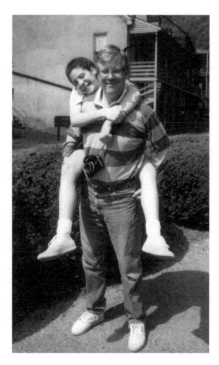

Here's Fred helping his daughter Elizabeth take a "load off" during a family outing in Harper's Ferry, West Virginia.

but everybody's overall pattern is different. I've known hundreds of people who stutter, and I have seen no two people who stutter alike.

When we begin to realize what these tricks are, and try to identify and monitor them, we begin to learn what stuttering actually is. The first phase of this was entirely a monitoring and identification phase, and it's a phase that I will continue to go through for quite a while. I'm always finding new things that I have done in the past but have buried under other tricks. People have talked about it as trying to peel an onion. You take off one of the outer layers and underneath that there's another trick, and underneath that, another one.

In my case, a lot of these tricks were learned in clusters. For instance, if I would lose eye contact, I would go into a very specific type of struggle pattern. But if I maintained eye contact, I would not usually employ any of those tricks. So if you identify one trick, and work on it, and it drops out of your speech, many others also drop out of your speech. For the first few months I was just monitoring these things. After very actively monitoring these tricks, many of them just dropped out on their own.

> I'm beginning to realize that stuttering is not really a speech problem, at least not one of speech production, because most people who stutter can speak perfectly fluently most of the time anyway. Stuttering is more of a fear problem.

After you monitor and catalogue all your tricks and get rid of a lot of them, you enter into a phase that they call open stuttering, which basically is just stuttering without any tricks at all. That's the hardest thing to do, and it's somewhat ugly because you are not trying to hide anything. Initially it is pretty uncomfortable, but it's a phase that you really need to go through, because if you try to speed it up too much, you tend to fall back into developing other tricks.

After a few months we began to go into the phase of voluntary stuttering. This consists of throwing in some false stuttering in your speech during periods of fluency, which appears, on the face of it, to be counter-productive, but really is not.

I'm beginning to realize that stuttering is not really a speech problem, at least not one of speech production, because most people who stutter can speak perfectly fluently most of the time anyway. Stuttering is more of a fear problem. The avoidances condition, or trigger, the fear, and the fear maintains our struggle. So, there is nothing we need to do to try to achieve fluency, directly, because fluency will come on its own. Fluency comes as a by-product of getting rid of all the avoidances and, consequently, fear of speaking.

It's absolutely the most effective approach I've ever tried. It's not so much achieving fluency as it is a loss of fear and becoming more comfortable as a result. In the last couple of years I have really increased my level of comfort in speaking, decreased most of my avoidances, and this has made a tremendous improvement in my quality of life. I am working toward being a more effective communicator, a person who does not avoid speaking situations because of stuttering and who wants to be more comfortable in his speech.

Group meetings have helped me a lot, too. I would encourage stutterers of all ages to get involved in groups like the ones associated with the National Stuttering Association. These meetings encourage me to not hide my stuttering.

Another worthwhile activity has been speaking to fluency disorders classes at local universities, and informing the speech pathology students what it's like to grow up being a person who stutters. I have spoken to classes at the University of Maryland and Gallaudet University, telling these students what it is really like to be a person who stutters, the problems we go through, and even all the bad, but well-intended, advice many of us have been given over the years.

> In the last couple of years I have really increased my level of comfort in speaking, decreased most of my avoidances, and this has made a tremendous improvement in my quality of life.

Author: Fred A. Lewis.

Fred is a fifty-five-year-old research scientist who works on schistosomiasis, one of the most prevalent infectious diseases in the tropics. He was born in Atlanta, Texas, and now lives in Gaithersburg, Maryland. He and his wife Maureen have been married for thirty years and have one son and one daughter. In what little spare time he has he enjoys reading, listening to classical music, and assisting in leading a local chapter of the National Stuttering Association.

407-001-TR-ST-001-2001

My Speech Difficulty
Led Me to Special Children

I AM A FORTY-FIVE-YEAR-OLD, MILD-TO-MODERATE STUTTERER WITH a bachelor's and a master's plus forty-eight credits in special education. Why do I teach special children? An incident led me to special education. This little guy was six, from an Hispanic family, and in special preschool. He didn't speak. He didn't make eye contact. The only human contact he made was when he knew that he was expected to go somewhere; he would stick one arm straight up in the air and curve his fingers and expect his companion to stick one arm straight down and curve his or her fingers into his. One companion was a Spanish-speaking college student who came in between classes. He was chosen with the hope that he could get the little boy to talk.

> It wasn't until I started working in special education that I realized I had a stuttering problem. My experience with speech difficulties wasn't new to me, just the notion that it was a problem shared by others.

One day the little boy and his student buddy were in the pool. The child was terrified of the water and would make his body go rigid. His companion would wade him around in an inflatable donut ring. One day he started to take the little boy out of the donut ring, and he accidentally dropped him down into the pool. A high pitch wail rang out. All of us sat there and looked at each other with tears in our eyes because that was the first sound we had ever heard from him. We finally believed that he could do something to let us know he was very unhappy. I always thought that if I could unlock and unleash potential, and find out what's "in there," it would be so rewarding and helpful. That's why I teach special children.

It wasn't until I started working in special education that I realized I had a stuttering problem. My experience with speech difficulties wasn't new to me, just the notion that it was a problem shared by others. I began to pay attention to it in some of the children and began to observe and hear it in my own speech. All the way through school, I had always noticed that if I were participating in a conversation, by the time I figured out my contribution and said my thing, people would look at me like, "We passed that a long time ago." I was pretty shy about talking in a group or in front of a group.

> I can be sitting there thinking and put my hands and fingertips together and kind of draw them apart as the sentence forms in my mind, and I can say it. This hand thing can really help.

I usually have to think things through in my mind or write them before I can say them. I can be sitting there thinking and put my hands and fingertips together and kind of draw them apart as the sentence forms in my mind, and I can say it. This hand thing can really help. There are still some pauses in my speech, but not a lot of repeats, just a lot of halting.

Nevertheless, I've done a lot of presentations to large groups—four to five hundred. One I'll never forget. I was director of Bible School, and I had to give out awards to the teachers and their helpers and do the little speech that you always do at the end of the term. I got up there and said, "Good evening." And it came out, *"Good evening,"* the pitch of my voice was lower, and I sounded almost sexy. My friend Phil had changed the mike and sound system around a little. So, I stopped and said, "Whew, Phil you make even me sound good." Then, I was ready to go. I did a pretty good job with that speech.

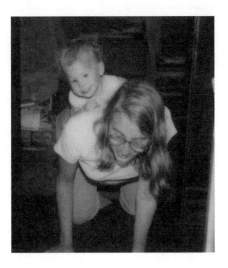

Verna giving one of her children a ride. Go faster, Mommy!

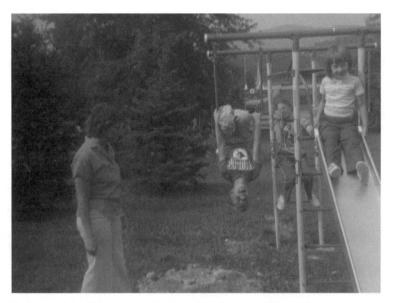

Verna supervises children at home, too. Here she watches her children perform various gymnastic stunts.

My stuttering has affected my career choice and still affects aspects of my job today. I never felt like getting certified in regular education just because I didn't want to talk in front of that many people at once. And I don't like to talk in front of groups of adults. When I have to, I really have to practice. I usually write everything down and practice it beforehand. I glance up to make eye contact every now and then and hold my paper tight with my thumb at my place so I won't lose my place. I read the whole thing very fast. I even used to encourage my daughter to practice school presentations. I would make her read her book reports over and over in front of the mirror and tape record them to see how they sounded.

As part of my job, I attend and present at Individualized Education Plan meetings. These are high-tension times for me. The first one I have with a parent I usually sound like an idiot just because it takes me so long to say the things I need to say. Thank goodness the forms are very structured and I can just plow through them with the parents. The tough meetings are the ones with the parent, the regular education teacher, the administrator, the speech therapist, the physical therapist, foster placement teams, and a half-dozen other agency representatives around the table. I'm sitting there thinking, "I don't want to talk to all these people at once. I don't want them all to hear me." Yet, I'm the authority. I have to and do talk to them all at once.

On the other hand, children are always easier for me. I remember the first year I taught I was scared to death. I had twelve children, kindergarten to third grade, and no aide. I put the kiddies in a circle on the floor and I sat down with them. I could read to them and do little activities out of the books with them. I would be comfortable and my knees wouldn't be knocking together. I'd have something structured to go by and I did pretty well.

Having a speech problem has also helped me as a special education teacher. It affects how I relate to the children. Children usually trust me. I have a friend who has a doctorate in special education who tells me that I could make a cat talk. Many times children look like they don't know things and they get skipped over a lot. I realize that it may take ten seconds for the child to process and get the answer out. Therefore, I cue the child that I'm going to ask a question, then I ask. I know that sometimes I have to draw the sentence in my head before I can answer, so I give them the same chance. I'm slow, and I understand if they are too.

I'm sitting there thinking, "I don't want to talk to all these people at once. I don't want them all to hear me." Yet, I'm the authority. I have to and do talk to them all at once.

Author: Verna Jane Corley.
Verna was born in Petersburg, West Virginia, and is now married with four children. She enjoys sewing, crocheting, and reading.

408-001-TR-ST-001-2001

My Wife
Made the Difference

I HAVE HAD BOTH GOOD AND BAD EXPERIENCES WITH MY STUTTERING during the course of my life. As a young child, I experienced more horrible instances than good ones, but as I matured good experiences began to appear more often.

My parents' reaction to my stuttering was very negative from the beginning. My fourth-grade teacher wrote a note to my parents about my speech trouble. My parents were very upset, and after a while both my teacher and my parents began fighting back and forth. That teacher was outstanding and finally convinced my parents to agree to send me to a speech therapist. But my parents were still very embarrassed about the whole darn thing. If someone would say something about the way that I talked, my mother's face would get very red. She blamed my stuttering on an experience that I had as a toddler. She said that I crawled over to my grandmother's mop that had bleach on it and started chewing on it. She thought that this left some scar tissue in my throat, but I do not think that incident had anything to do with it. I think my mother was looking for something to blame it on.

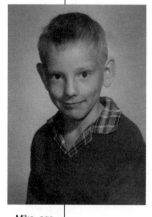

Mike, age six, at the beginning of his school experience with stuttering.

Aside from affecting my family members' perceptions of me, I also struggled with my stuttering problem at school. I don't think that teachers knew how to deal with it. In my case, the teacher

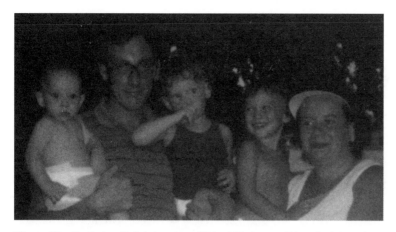

Mike and his wife, Susie, with their three sons, Michael, Matthew, and Marc. Susie helped Mike achieve the self-confidence he needed to control his stuttering.

kind of overlooked me; I kind of got stuck back in the corner. I think if a kid doesn't grasp certain things, they just get more and more lost. I think being overlooked affected my reading because I had to use the little bit that I picked up in class to teach myself.

Bad experiences with teachers continued even until the eighth and ninth grades. I recall once when I had a permission slip to get into my locker between classes because I had a doctor's appointment. A teacher came out and asked me what I was doing at my locker. I was trying to tell him, but because I was very upset, I couldn't tell him. He grabbed me and started slamming me into my locker. I tried to fight him because he was hurting me, and he tore my shirt off my back. He then dragged me up the steps to the principal's office, and I was expelled from school for three days. Teachers were not prepared to deal with this type of thing back in the sixties and seventies. I see now that teachers try very hard to deal with stuttering. I just wish that they knew more when I went to school.

Another time, when I was seventeen, I was driving down the road and I ran a red light. I got pulled over by a police officer and he started asking me questions. I started to stutter. He took me into the city building because he thought I was drinking. These are the kinds of things that you go through as a stutterer. You have to have a great sense of humor. Today, I just laugh.

She blamed my stuttering on an experience that I had as a toddler. She said that I crawled over to my grandmother's mop that had bleach on it and started chewing on it.

I have encountered a lot of people who have been rude about my stuttering, but I've also met a lot of nice people. I do consulting for a company in Philadelphia. One day I walked into their conference room to meet the president of the company. He started talking and he had a lot of trouble saying a lot of words. The guy that I worked for got me and the president off to ourselves, and explained to this man that I stuttered too. He told me that life is what you make of it. He told me that he was told that he couldn't do a lot of things and that made him work even more.

My stuttering has never held me back. In fact, there has never been a person I've met who after a while, I didn't win his or her confidence. It is the people who are afraid to deal with the stuttering that turn away. You'll start talking to them and you'll have trouble saying words. They will turn their head and not listen because they are afraid to look you in the face.

Growing up I really did experience a wide variety of reactions from people who heard my stuttering. Even kids will make fun of kids. I was called all kinds of names. But, I think it makes you a better person in the long run. I also made a lot of friends talking the way that I do. At one place of work, I was a very popular guy. I felt that people didn't go behind my back and say things. It might have taken me a couple of minutes more to tell somebody what to do, but people laughed with me, not at me. When I began working at a different plant, I got called names. I was called "crazy lips" and "stutter box." But, I don't care about name-calling because it only makes them look bad, not me.

I once did not get a job because of my stuttering. I went for a job interview to sell tires. The interviewer said, "Do you talk this way all of the time?" I said, "Yeah," and he said that he didn't think that I was capable of doing the job. I was able to do the job, but I stuttered so badly that he thought it would interfere with my performance. Later, when I did get my first decent job for another company, I worked really hard. I eventually became

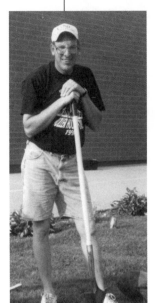

Mike, planting a sign at his local elementary school.

When I began working at a different plant, I got called names. I was called "crazy lips" and "stutter box." But, I don't care about name-calling because it only makes them look bad, not me.

a supervisor, which people never thought I could do. I had as many as forty-seven people working under me, all trained by me. So, I think that there is hope for people who talk the way that I do.

I attribute much of my success to my wife, Susie, who has really helped me out a lot. I think it is because I feel comfortable around her. That makes a big difference. Back when I first met Susie, I stuttered very badly while talking to people. After dating Susie and being around her and her mother for about six months, I started to improve. Susie's mother and Susie helped me so much. They always made me feel comfortable. They weren't ashamed to eat out in a restaurant with me. Their acceptance was much different than what I was used to. My family treated me like I had a horrible disease. Meeting and getting to know Susie, I was treated like a person. Life was great. I gained the confidence necessary to control my stuttering.

> I attribute a lot of my success to my wife, Susie, who has really helped me out a lot. I think it is because I feel comfortable around her.

Author: Michael Keith Baker.
Mike is an animal control officer, guitar player, singer, fisherman, and hunter from Moundsville, West Virginia. In addition to his work and hobbies, he is a husband of twenty-four years and a father of three wonderful boys. Mike has never viewed his stuttering as a handicap. Instead, he stresses that any door that has been closed because of his stuttering wasn't worth going through.

409-001-TR-ST-001-2001

"Think Positive"

I'M FIFTY-FIVE YEARS OLD NOW AND I HAVE STUTTERED SINCE THE the age of three. When I was three, my mother was expecting, but my parents didn't tell me that she was pregnant. I didn't realize it. When my mother had my younger brother, my father took me to the hospital and asked me how I liked my baby brother. I was so shocked that I didn't utter a sound for six months. My parents took me to the doctor to find out what the problem was. He just said that the birth of my little brother was a shock to me and that I would eventually start talking again. When I began to talk again, I stuttered. I didn't stammer; I stuttered and have continued to stutter ever since.

> When my mother had my younger brother, my father took me to the hospital and asked me how I liked my baby brother. I was so shocked that I didn't utter a sound for six months.

When I was about six years old, my parents took me to the University of Pittsburgh to a clinic at the Cathedral of Learning. I had all kinds of hearing and speech tests. They checked everything and said that there was nothing wrong with me physically and that I would probably outgrow it by the age of twelve. I didn't. I had speech lessons every Friday afternoon starting in first grade. I would go for an hour or a half-hour speech lesson. I remember learning things like how to pant like a dog to control my breathing, and taking my thumb and rubbing it on my palm to distract my thinking.

A lot of my problem was in my head, something with my mind related to a younger brother that I had no idea was coming.

My parents never told me until I was older that I also had an older brother who died at birth. I think a lot of my stuttering was mental.

I had strategies. I would come to words in conversation, such as my name, that I couldn't say, and I would rearrange the sentence. I could say the word in another sentence form and many times I would just substitute the words. That would help me a lot. But, it is hard to do sometimes. You have to think fast. We used to think that one of my problems was that I was trying to say words faster than my brain was putting them in there for me to speak. I don't know if that was it or not, but that is what someone told me years ago was one of my problems.

My wife was expecting, and I wanted to join the service and be a pilot. I couldn't pass the test to be a pilot because I stuttered.

I flunked several classes in high school and college. I took Latin I and II and had to stand up and recite, which I could not do. I didn't even like getting up in front of a group and talking in high school. We had to learn poems and stand up and say them. I couldn't do it. I still avoid these types of situations today, but I can read aloud to children without a problem. Not too long ago, I visited an elementary school for Dr. Seuss Day. They gave me a book, I introduced myself to the third-grade class, and I read. They had no idea that I stuttered, so I didn't have a problem.

Also, while in college, I had two years of ROTC, Reserve Officers Training Corps, for the service. My wife was expecting, and I wanted to join the service and be a pilot. I couldn't pass the test to

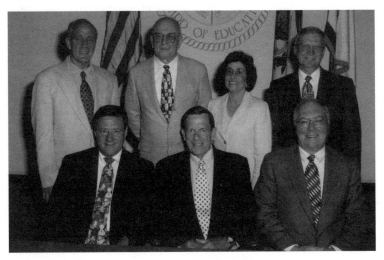

Doug, seated at left, takes his place on the Board of Education.

be a pilot because I stuttered. If I hadn't stuttered, I would probably be flying. I am flying today; but back then, I stuttered too bad to even fly. So that held me back.

Stuttering used to greatly affect my social interactions. I remember that when I was little, I was withdrawn. Also, when

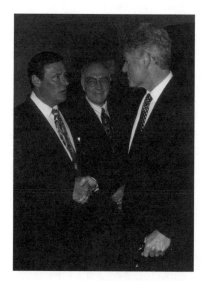

President Clinton meets Doug Gray at his local high school during President Clinton's town hall meeting.

I was younger, there were a lot of times when I would just stand back and not even enter into a conversation. And, at parties and a lot of things at school I didn't participate because I stuttered. But usually with friends, the guys and girls I hung around with, I didn't stutter because I knew them and they knew me.

Today, I am an insurance agent with Nationwide Insurance. I have to talk to people on the telephone and in person about their insurance, about their problems, and everything else. I have gained the confidence to be able to do that. I don't have that much of a problem with my stuttering anymore, if I get my rest. If I don't, I do stutter. If I sleep in some mornings to make up for any lost time, I do fine.

Since being so withdrawn and introverted in high school and college, I have pursued many leadership positions. Later in my career at Jaycees, I gathered the courage to run for the president position, and I got it. Since then, I have become involved in several organizations. I was president of the Strawberry Festival, and I am on the school board now. I've been President of the Shrine Club and about four or five other organizations. Anything I'm in, I put everything into it. I have given many talks in front of people in these organizations and have done quite well.

I recently became involved in real estate and have been teaching at Fairmont State College. I now like teaching and talking in front of a group. I overcame my stuttering. I did it over time, but it took me a long time to do it. I had to get in a situation that made me stop stuttering and that was my job. I have to talk to people every day.

You can always help yourself. You can always improve. There are so many new things today that were not available when I was young. Your teachers can help you more than anything can. With the new improvements and the different therapy techniques for stuttering, you can change yourself. If you listen to your teachers and they say you need to practice, go ahead and practice. If you don't, no one else can stop it for you. You have to want to do it yourself. If you don't work with them or do the techniques, you will keep stuttering from now on.

I don't have that much of a problem with my stuttering anymore, if I get my rest. If I don't, I do stutter. If I sleep in some morning to make up for any lost time, I do fine.

You have to think positive. I've taken all sorts of classes for positive thinking that helped me. It is up to the stutterer. You can do it if you want to. With the techniques and the learning tools, change is out there for you. It might not be tomorrow, it might not be today, but it is coming for you.

Author: Paul Douglas Gray.
Doug is an insurance agent and real estate owner in Clarksburg, West Virginia. He is the proud father of four and grandfather of six. Doug enjoys West Virginia football and holding leadership roles within the community: vice president of the Harrison County Board of Education, a past president of the Clarksburg Lions, a member of Central West Virginia Shrine Club, Clarksburg Life Underwriters, The West Virginia Strawberry Festival, and the Board of Directors of the Morgantown Touchdown Club.

410-001-TR-ST-001-2001

The Red Rabbit
Ran 'Round the Room

Wᴇᴇᴋ ᴀꜰᴛᴇʀ ᴡᴇᴇᴋ ɪ ʟᴏᴏᴋᴇᴅ ᴜᴘ ꜰʀᴏᴍ ᴍʏ ɢʀᴀᴅᴇ-sᴄʜᴏᴏʟ ᴅᴇsᴋ when I heard the speech therapist call out my name. Feeling slightly awkward, I would get up and follow her, and think to myself that there was no point to the things that she asked me to do while out of class. As a young child, I saw no benefit in sitting around a table with other kids (some that I did know and a few that I did not) and repeating phrases like "the red rabbit ran around the room." Plus, my stuttering really didn't bother me that much. I always felt that I could speak fairly well when I had to.

According to my mother and father, I became nonverbal after hospitalization for rheumatic fever at age four. Apparently, when I started to talk again, I talked real fast, and they used to tell me things like, "slow down," "take your time," and "think what you're going to say." From what they told me, that's about the time the stuttering started.

During my junior high school years we moved to Indiana. Within a few weeks into the school year, I was called out of my classroom by the assistant principal and told I would be enrolled in therapy once again. During these sessions, we merely sat and talked. I don't recall learning any fluency skills from that therapist either. I think I was one of those kids who was probably quite fluent when

> According to my mother and father, I became nonverbal after hospitalization for rheumatic fever at age four. Apparently, when I started to talk again, I talked real fast, and they used to tell me things like, "slow down," "take your time," and "think what you're going to say."

I was in the clinic room, and so there probably really was not a whole lot that he could do for me.

Although my disfluency problem was obvious enough to be again referred for therapy, I did not think of my speech as being that much of a problem. I recall that when I was in fifth or sixth grade, my family bought a tape recorder for Christmas. After the holidays had settled in, we listened to the tapes, some with me speaking. I was amazed at how disfluent I sounded. Yet, I figured I would just wake up one morning and speak fluently.

The hard realizations of the possible effects of my stuttering did not occur until about my senior year in high school, I think in English class. While attempting to answer a question that the teacher posed, I encountered a fairly long block. Laughter rose like a wave through the classroom. I realized that if people who had known me for three, four, or even five years would laugh at me, college and its new experiences could become a nightmare.

Because of this experience, I became embarrassed about my speech for the first time in my life. I began avoiding social situations and tried to hide my disfluencies. I also started to use imprecise language while avoiding words that I knew I might stutter on. I often referred to people during conversation as "what's-his-name," making conversation awkward.

I really worked hard to hide my stuttering, and the harder I tried to hide it the worse the problem became. Concerns about my disfluency consumed my life. My awareness really did increase as I got older. And the problem was that as I got more aware, I didn't have any skills. I didn't have the skills to fall back on to be able to change things. I felt like whatever happened, happened, and there was no way that I could change it.

After graduation, I went to college with the fear of becoming an object of humiliation. I did not talk to people. I avoided meeting people and I became very surly and introverted. I registered for large classes instead of small ones. Becoming a number rather than a name comforted me. My grades reflected my obsession with

> After the holidays had settled in we listened to the tapes, some with me speaking. I was amazed at how disfluent I sounded. Yet, I figured I would just wake up one morning and speak fluently.

> After graduation, I went to college with the fear of becoming an object of humiliation. I did not talk to people. I avoided meeting people and I became very surly and introverted.

becoming an outsider. With poor grades, I quit school for a year and went to work in a factory.

Taking that year off in life helped me get a grasp once again on my goals in life. During this time I chose to continue my education to become a speech-language pathologist. Changing my major to speech and hearing seemed like the logical thing to do. While learning about speech and speaking, I evolved as a speaker myself and gained a lot of knowledge about my own speech deficiency.

With my newly found major, I also decided to begin therapy again. This therapy helped me much more than ever before. At this time, I was ready to admit to my attitudes and behaviors, and I worked to change them. By learning to conquer my own fears of failure, I found that I could speak much better than I ever thought I would in situations that I had previously avoided.

Deciding to become a professional in the field of speech and language became one of the smartest things that I have ever done. I am now a professor and the Director of the Program in Communication Sciences and Disorders at Western Illinois University. As an educator, clinician, researcher, and stutterer, I've had ample opportunity to consider the age-old question of what causes stuttering. At the core of the problem is a breakdown in the stutterer's speech. This can have many causes and separates

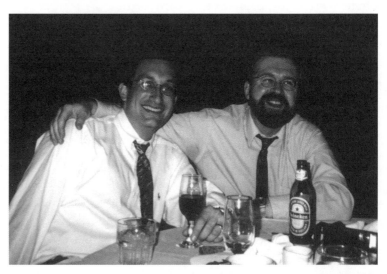

Bob Quesal, on the right, with friend and colleague Scott Yaruss at the June 2000 National Stuttering Association convention in Chicago.

stutterers into many subtypes. Some stutterers have motor problems, while others battle a more language-based disfluency, for example.

On top of the core problem, the child or adult then collects experiences as a stutterer and adds on psychological problems, such as coping behaviors, avoidances, and ineffective ways of coping. This psychological baggage makes the problem worse.

There's a related analogy I've found helpful in considering my stuttering: If you watch people walking in the snow who are confident, they are not really worried about falling and they walk normally. People who are worried about falling walk more tenuously. They are not walking in a normal way.

> Other children may be more vulnerable, more sensitive, and probably have a more difficult time dealing with their problems.

The kids who have been tensely walking in the snow their entire lives have developed their own way of dealing with their speech differences and they worry about it. These are the types of things that cause children to develop psychological baggage at a young age. Kids who outgrow stuttering may not be very bothered by their disfluencies, and as they mature, their problems smooth out. Other children may be more vulnerable, more sensitive, and probably have a more difficult time dealing with their problems.

A stutterer must learn not to avoid, not to hold negative attitudes, and not to withdraw as I once did. Only then can a stutterer walk in the snow without worrying about falling.

Author: Robert W. Quesal.
Bob is forty-eight and a college professor in Macomb, Illinois. He was born in Yonkers, New York, and is married with two children. Bob feels that his story is one of many and doesn't pretend to be like all stutterers. Bob likes reading, sports, and pre-Beatles rock.

411-001-TR-ST-001-2001

I Thought
I Was the Only One

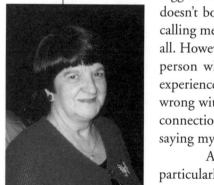

Alta Sliger.

I HAVE KIND OF ACCEPTED THE FACT THAT I DO STUTTER. But, I still have some things that bother me. I think one of my biggest difficulties has to do with the telephone. It doesn't bother me calling my friends or my friends calling me. A person calling me doesn't bother me at all. However, when I call someone and try to tell the person who I am, I have a really hard time. I've experienced people saying, "Oh, is there something wrong with your phone?" or "Maybe we have a bad connection." It is not that, I am just having trouble saying my name or something.

Another situation that bothers me particularly is when I first meet someone and they do not know that I stutter. It is kind of hard because they feel uncomfortable. It does pose a problem. It doesn't bother me that much, but I think, "Gee, how is it going to affect them? How are they going to perceive me?"

One typical reaction to my stuttering really infuriates me. They say, "Oh, honey, just slow down and take your time." A few people also try to finish my sentences for me. Of course, I'm just stubborn enough that even if they finish my sentence for me, I go ahead and finish it myself—no matter how long it takes.

For the most part, though, people have been very understanding and kind. They seem to accept it. People that I first meet are usually very gracious. But, after I leave, I don't know what they may say about me. It isn't really like this so much now, but back in high school the people who didn't know that I stuttered had a first reaction to laugh. You know how teenagers are; they don't know any different.

There have been some negative experiences like these, but my stuttering has also resulted in some positive things in my life. For example, I have become more understanding of people's disabilities or handicaps. I am probably more compassionate than I would've been if I didn't have the stuttering problem. I think I might have the tendency to be kind of a snob to other people with disabilities if I didn't have my own problem.

Of course, I'm just stubborn enough that even if they finish my sentence for me, I go ahead and finish it myself—no matter how long it takes.

I also think that stuttering has given me a reason to avoid the things that I do not want to do anyway, things that I otherwise would not have been able to get out of easily. For example, we sometimes have trouble electing officers for the social sorority that I belong to. Everyone says, "I can't do it. I don't want to do it. I don't have time." And they get coaxed into it. No one expects me to do it because they know I stutter. Stuttering has given me an excuse for not doing things that I really don't want to do anyway. I think everyone tries to find an excuse for things they don't want to do, and stuttering has been my excuse.

I think probably back in high school stuttering may have hindered my participation in things like school plays. Possibly if I had not stuttered, I would have participated more; but, I cannot say for sure. I have always thought it would be neat to take part in a play or something, but then I would have had to memorize all of those lines. Really, I don't know if it would have been something that I would have done if I had not stuttered.

I do feel like stuttering has not affected my career. My job has always been very satisfactory to me. I have enjoyed sitting down and keeping a set of books, doing payroll, and performing secretarial duties. My job now really fits me to a "T"—it's perfect because I work strictly with a computer system. I kind of work on my own and at my own pace. The other girls in the office have to wait on the public. They have to answer the phone so they cannot devote their entire day to their work. I don't have to deal with the public in person or by phone, and that makes it nice.

Stuttering really hasn't affected my social life either. I belong to a bridge club and a social sorority. I am a member of the Board of Directors for Main Street Kingwood. I haven't let it hold me back much. For the most part, I do what I want to do. Maybe if I didn't stutter I would want to do different things. I may have adjusted my life to recognize my shortcomings. I know that there are things that I don't do. I won't say that I can't do them. I don't want to do them because I stutter. But, really for the most part I do the things that I want to do, even if that does sound a little contradictory. I think that if I didn't stutter there might be more things that I might want to do, but I don't know because I have never experienced not stuttering. So, I don't know that I would do anything different.

> ...but my stuttering has also resulted in some positive things in my life. For example, I have become more understanding of people's disabilities or handicaps. I am probably more compassionate than I would've been if I didn't have the stuttering problem.

I always stuttered growing up. I didn't have any therapy until I graduated from high school and started in the Career College. The head of the Career College told me about the speech program at the university. Prior to that time, I didn't know that there was anything you could do about stuttering. I came from a small town, and no one stuttered around me, so I didn't know. I mean, heck, I just did not know that there were people who stuttered besides me.

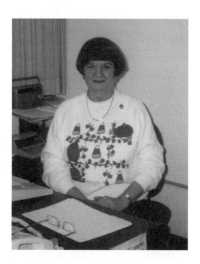

Alta dressed for Halloween at the office. Candy, anyone?

As I have discussed with my therapist, therapy sometimes makes my stuttering situation really frustrating for me. When I am having formal therapy I can control my stuttering very, very well. The real frustrating part is that I cannot maintain my fluency outside of therapy. It makes me question why it is like this when I am not having therapy. It seems to me that it should be that once you have the therapy, you are cured. Of course you aren't, but you go for a period of time fluent and then gradually you are reverting, and then all of a sudden here you are, stuttering again really bad!

Group therapy sessions have been very beneficial to me. I have become acquainted with other people who stutter. It has really helped me to know that there are others who have experienced the same things, the same frustrations that I have experienced. It is always nice to know that you are not struggling alone. There are other people who have the same struggles.

I really think that speech therapists need to understand and be aware of a stutterer's feelings. A speech therapist who does not stutter probably doesn't have a clue as to how people who stutter feel. I hope I can help speech therapists and aspiring students understand.

Author: Alta F. Sliger.

Alta is a data entry clerk at the Preston County Assessor's Office and was previously employed for thirty years as clerk-secretary for the West Virginia Northern Railroad Company. A native Prestonian, she has resided in Kingwood for the past forty-five years. Alta is active in her community and social sorority and enjoys playing bridge. Her hobbies are reading, traveling, and socializing with friends.

412-001-TR-ST-001-2001

The head of the Career College told me about the speech program at the university. Prior to that time I didn't know that there was anything you could do about stuttering. I came from a small town, and no one stuttered around me, so I didn't know.

I Didn't Want to Be Different

ACKNOWLEDGING THAT I STUTTERED TOOK INCREDIBLE courage. And it took years. At twenty-one I was finally able to admit to myself and others that I stuttered. I was a college student and seeing a school psychologist. In the fourth session I told the psychologist that I was a "person who stuttered." It was then that I began to own my stuttering. My "admission" is what I needed to do in order to take the first step toward forging a new and more fulfilled Michael.

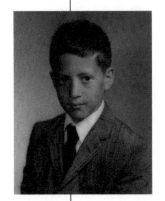

Michael circa 1960.

Until then, my stuttering represented my entire self-image. I was dominated by my stuttering. It was difficult for me to express my wants and feelings. I stuttered and worried about what the listener would think of me as a person who stuttered. I struggled to push words out and felt helpless, anxious, afraid, shamed, and guilty. When words emerged, I questioned myself: was I saying what I really meant, or was I just using words I could be fluent on, regardless of whether or not they truly expressed my intentions? I learned how to disguise my stuttering, hiding it in various ways. Often this meant substituting words that were easier to say.

I became an expert at avoiding verbal communications. I dealt with many everyday situations in silence. I would point to what I wanted on the menu in restaurants. I asked family members or friends to buy the ticket for a movie or concert; if I had to do it, I'd use gestures as much as possible, my fingers, for example, indicating how many tickets I wanted. I answered questions by nodding or shaking my head. I didn't speak unless it was absolutely necessary. I'd try to let a short simple "yes" or "no" suffice. I even avoided people because they reminded me that I was unable to communicate verbally.

In the first and second grades, I remember being placed in the "slow class." I played with blocks a lot. When I read out loud, I stuttered. Fortunately, a reading teacher eventually asked me to read silently and answer questions about what I had read. I did fine and was mainstreamed back into my peer group class.

When I was in the third grade, a yellow "speech card" was placed on the blackboard chalk ledge every Wednesday to remind me to go to speech therapy. The card also served as a silent reminder that I was different. I often walked out sheepishly from class and tried to hide in the bathroom. The school speech therapist worked on my "s" and "th" sounds, but never talked about my stuttering or how I felt.

Throughout my school years, I recall using tricks to enable me to get through class presentations despite my blocks, blinking eyes, and head-jerking tension. These strategies were many and varied: talking in a low voice, talking very fast, nodding my head, and using filler words. I remember doing a talk on Copernicus in eighth grade. That day the word "okay" was my prop; I inserted it after almost every word. Without doubt, my grades suffered because of my stuttering.

Other childhood memories involve my mother's constant advice to, "Stop. Think before you speak," and the ulcer I developed in the third and again in the seventh grade. Eating out at restaurants was torture. Waiters would mimic my stuttering when I tried to order. I resorted to ordering cheeseburgers instead of a hamburger—what I really wanted—for sixteen years of my life because it was easier for me to say.

After high school, I did a lot of study and research about stuttering. I read numerous articles, in search of answers and,

In the first and second grades, I remember being placed in the "slow class." I played with blocks a lot.

Throughout my school years, I recall using tricks to enable me to get through class presentations despite my blocks, blinking eyes, and head-jerking tension. These strategies were many and varied: talking in a low voice, talking very fast, nodding my head, and using filler words.

hopefully, my cure. It was towards the end of this quest that I met with the university psychologist and started to really talk about my life and my stuttering. The psychologist recommended speech therapy. I followed through and began speech therapy for the third time in my life. This time, however, it was different. With therapeutic guidance, I began a year-and-a-half process of self-disclosure, discovery, practice, and ultimately, liberation.

> **With therapeutic guidance, I began a year-and-a-half process of self-disclosure, discovery, practice, and ultimately, liberation.**

I began to see how I used my stuttering as an excuse. It let me legitimize my lack of effort, interest, and aspirations. I felt that I couldn't participate fully in life because I stuttered, and so embraced an attitude of "Why assert myself?" The pursuit and development of interests, goals, and relationships had no place in my life, I figured. I felt ambivalence toward my parents and thought no one would marry me because I stuttered. Regarding academics, I was afraid to ask a question despite my thirst for knowledge and answers. And when I considered employment and a career, I couldn't imagine a profession that would not demand verbal faculty.

The speech therapist helped me look at past events that led me to assume the identity of "stutterer." I realized I needed to re-create myself, and with guidance, I was successful. Breaking away from my past was key. For me, this meant giving up the idea that I was a person who was unable to express feelings and desires without stuttering, and it meant trying to understand the behavior controlling me. For example, I noted how my stuttering seemed to worsen when I spoke of my family or myself. Gradually, I became less and less afraid of verbal communication, and more willing to take risks, speaking and otherwise.

> **At first I hated listening to myself and being reminded of how I spoke. However, in time, the tape recorder became less of an enemy and more of an ally in my journey.**

I know that stuttering—its cause, patterns, and effects—is not the same for everybody. In my case, looking back, I know it was important that I objectified my stuttering behavior. This involved separating myself from a destructive self-concept and assuming a liberating self-concept.

As for the more technical side of my speech therapy, I spent hours working with a tape recorder. With the recorder on, I practiced reading from books, monologue, and conversation. At first I hated listening to myself and being reminded of how I spoke. However, in time, the tape recorder became less of an enemy and more of an ally in my journey.

Greatly inspired by my experience, I became involved in something incredibly important. One evening in 1976, a group of clinicians and clients from the University of California Santa Barbara Speech Clinic went out for dinner to celebrate the end of the term. I was sitting with five other people who stuttered and had also been in speech therapy.

While we were trying to have a relaxing conversation, the clinicians sat there counting our disfluencies. I decided to get up and move to another table. The rest of the people who stuttered joined me. That night in Santa Barbara, California, we formed the nation's first stuttering self-help group. Later that year, I met Bob Goldman and together we started the National Stuttering Project. Now known as the National Stuttering Association, it has over 2,700 members and self-help groups meeting in more than seventy-five cities around the country. Dealing with my stuttering and building bonds with other people who stutter has enriched my life tremendously.

Author: Michael Sugarman.
Michael is father to his ten-year-old daughter, Rebekah, and husband to Kim for fourteen years. He is a medical social worker from Oakland, California, and enjoys backpacking, gardening, and cooking. Michael co-founded the National Stuttering Association in 1977 and has been inducted into the National Stuttering Hall of Fame. He also received the first Consumer Award of Distinction by the International Fluency Association. Michael initiated the concept of an "International Stuttering Awareness Day" (ISAD) for the twenty-second of October. In 1998 he was the co-coordinator of the first ISAD On-Line Conference.

413-001-TR-ST-001-2001

And the Winner Is...

For FIFTY-NINE YEARS IT HAS BEEN AN EPIC STRUGGLE between two unyielding foes. A battle between light and darkness, between hope and resignation, between elation and despair. In the beginning it was a war between a bewildered and overmatched five-year-old child and a mysterious and merciless all-powerful opponent. In the child's corner were his parents who would have done anything to free their first born from the grasp of the adversary. But unknowing they hindered his escape by applying unbreakable chains so that any chance the child had to be victorious was taken away. The rather gifted child, the pride of his parents, was handicapped with a yoke he could not escape.

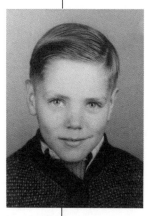

Larry in the 1940s.

One day when the child was in the woods with his dad he saw some wild grapes they called "bullesis." While showing them to his dad, he stumbled over the word, saying bul-bul-bul-bullesis. His dad, with a curious look on his face asked, what did you say? The child again attempted to say the word, but this time trying to control his speech began to strain and had an even harder time. And thus the fight between freedom (of speech) and slavery (to stuttering) was joined, a battle in which no separation or quarters can be given and can only end with one survivor.

The child has fought this strange malady from that moment until now with great courage and hope. For the first fourteen years, he was on his own. Teachers, friends, and relatives would give advice that at best was neutral. When he was nineteen, he saw a speech therapist in conjunction with a psychiatrist for a semester or two. Very little if any permanent value came from this therapy. Based on that experience, he concluded outside help would be of no benefit and that if he were to conquer stuttering, it was up to him. It would be twenty-nine more years before he again sought professional help.

When out of sight and sound of others, the child had no difficulty dispatching the enemy. And therein lay the mystery of the struggle and the hope for complete victory. Why? Why would the child have a silver tongue when alone and a broken tongue in the presence of others, even when the others were loving, supportive friends and family? For many years the child tried to solve this frustrating riddle.

The child, when alone, would play the role of an orator, trying to find the key to transferring the perfect fluency in private to the fluency he dreamed of having in public. But all attempts to exhibit the same smooth flowing speech in the presence of others, that was so easily and naturally available in private, always ended with frustration and the question, why can't I do it? The easy uninterrupted speech when by himself kept the hope alive that normal fluency in the presence of others would be achieved. He prayed every night that he would find the way out of the mire and never doubted that he would scale the "Cliffs of Impossibility."

In all other areas, the child was a winner. In grade school he was a leader, he was the strongest and fastest, and against whom all new kids were measured. After he was the only one in his seventh grade class to solve a riddle posed by the teacher, she said, if she had ever known a genius, it was he. He was a happy child. His speech didn't bother him until he tried to speak. In school, a daily example of this was his extreme difficulty in making his presence known when answering the class roll call.

His athleticism, leadership, and likable qualities continued to shine in high school where he was senior class president, valedictorian, and was voted Most Likely to Succeed, Best All Around, Most Industrious, and Most Dependable by his classmates. Full-page pictures of him for each of these honors were shown in the school yearbook. He was also still the fastest and strongest. His valedictory address is an experience he will always remember. He had never been able to speak before a crowd without great difficulty. He worked on the speech for weeks and prayed continuously that he would be fluent when giving it. He knew it by heart and gave it flawlessly before the packed auditorium, as he had numerous times when no one but him could hear. People were amazed and told him that he had conquered his stuttering. If only that had been true! But it was wonderful to have been fluent for that important occasion. That experience showed that fluent speech in public was possible for him and reinforced his belief that his goal would be achieved.

His college experiences were good but his speech remained bad. He had the most trouble when asking for laboratory equipment and supplies. He received his bachelor's and master's degrees in chemical engineering from Georgia Tech and his Ph.D. degree in chemical engineering from West Virginia University. He was a member of the freshman track and cross-country teams but because of late chemistry labs, stopped competing in these sports after his freshman year. His name was placed on the field house record board when he broke the Georgia Tech pushup record. One notable academic achievement was in a physics class of sixty-nine students, where he was the only one with a grade above 90.

I was that child, and after coming to West Virginia in 1962, I struggled on my own to achieve the fluency I wanted but gained no lasting success. In late spring of 1984, I was having a very hard time trying to talk. My speech was terrible and I could not make it better. I tried forcing my way through blocks only to exacerbate the problem. The only way for me not to stutter severely was to keep quiet. My many years of praying for help were answered on the radio by way of an Easter Seals announcement concerning speech therapy. After hearing this announcement, I went to the WVU hospital to see what they could offer. They recommended that I go to the WVU Department of Speech Pathology and Audiology. Shortly after the radio announcement, a second and equally important event occurred when I saw Joseph Sheehan, a speech therapist at UCLA, on a TV talk show. I was impressed with him and ordered his book, *Stuttering: Research and Therapy*. The WVU Speech Clinic and the insight gained from Sheehan's book put me on the pathway to fluency.

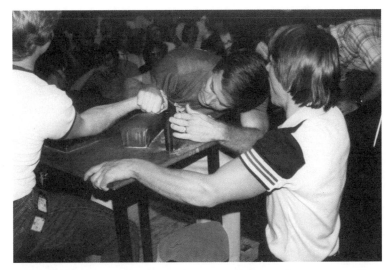

And the winner is Larry in a 1982 arm-wrestling contest. He has won the state arm-wrestling championships six times in West Virginia and once in Virginia.

When I started going to the clinic in June of 1984, I stuttered severely. At one of the early sessions, I found a "pot of gold" at the end of a rainbow. This pot of gold was fluency in reading. Lucia, my first student therapist, asked me to read something for her. Before going to the clinic, I had as much or more difficulty in reading as in speaking. The material I was asked to read described the physics of the rainbow and the legends and explanations people have used to explain the phenomenon. To my surprise and exhilaration, I was able to read the page-long article with very little trouble. It was gratifying to find that this discovered in-clinic reading fluency carried over to out-of-clinic situations. Being able to read fluently was a milestone in my therapy. I was elated over this success and it gave me confidence to build upon to make progress in my conversational speech.

> Being able to read fluently was a milestone in my therapy. I was elated over this success and it gave me confidence to build upon to make progress in my conversational speech.

And My Pathway to Victory Is...

Still missing a few road signs and is full of obstacles but has become less mysterious. The identified obstacles are an approach-avoidance conflict, a self-role conflict, and a false-role disorder. The approach-avoidance conflict is when I am undecided about going ahead or holding back. The self-role conflict is a speaker-listener disorder, which depends on how I perceive myself in relation to my listener or audience. My speech varies greatly with my audience and the social situation. I have a false-role disorder when I pretend not to be a stutterer.

Regardless of what initiated my stuttering, I believe my stuttering pattern is something that has been learned and is perpetuated by fear. When I struggle, I am trying to conceal my stuttering and when I hesitate because of a feared word or block with no sound, I am trying to avoid or deny my stuttering. If I am to achieve natural fluency, I must be expressive and not repressive. Not knowing how much difficulty I will have in a speaking situation and straining to be fluent are major causes of the anxiety which exacerbates my stuttering. When I can stutter smoothly, openly, and forward without shame, and be comfortable in both the stuttering mode and the fluency mode, I will be on my way to scaling the "Cliffs of Impossibility."

Achieving fluency in a low stress environment is no big deal and provides only an illusion of progress and "false hope."

My search for fluency can be titled, "Just Around the Corner." For me, the elusive fluency seems to have always been just around the corner. Since talking is so easy for almost everyone, and

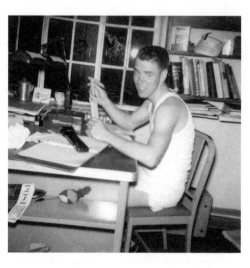

Larry in college circa 1960, no doubt studying. Note the slide rule. Is that a track suit he's wearing?

for me a good bit of the time, the positive reinforcement of complete fluency for extended periods has fueled the hope and expectation that the discovery of a simple key will open the gate to smooth flowing speech. On many important occasions, I have had near perfect fluency. People who know me look upon these occurrences as miraculous events, but they just reinforce my belief that I will achieve normal fluency.

After years of wondering, I now understand why I am 100 percent fluent in some situations but have great difficulty speaking in others. Achieving fluency in a low stress environment is no big deal and provides only an illusion of progress and "false hope." When my confidence is high and there is no fear, as when I am alone or in a relaxed situation, there is no stuttering. I believe my quest for consistent fluency will be achieved indirectly as a by-product of reducing my fear or by diminishing its effect on my speech.

Over the years, I have had false hope for a major break-through many times. These exciting discoveries, however, were not sufficient to put me over the top but were just necessary pieces of a bigger puzzle. Finally, I believe that I do have enough pieces of the puzzle to escape this web of frustration. Yet, until I catch the tiger (have sustainable fluent speech), my recipe for tiger stew (my plan for scaling the cliffs) will not be a prize winner. I may have the road map, but if I don't have enough courage and capacity to complete the journey, it will be of little use to me. To have free-flowing speech, I must break my ingrained stuttering habit of reacting to fear and conflict by holding back. To be free from its awesome power, I must sacrifice the comfort and safety of avoidance, and embrace the embarrassment of letting go and fully showing my stuttering. The often-heard advice to "go ahead and spit it out" seems to be valid after all. But, habits must be changed before that can be done.

There are many ways into the maze called stuttering and probably as many or more ways out of this thicket of entanglement. My attempts to find the way out of the morass has been a roller coaster tumultuous ride resulting in the greatest challenge in my life. My quest for fluent speech is a multiple-pronged challenge. In some speaking situations, I am at or near the summit, whereas in others I am still at the foot of the cliffs.

Some people may pity the poor person who stutters. But I'm glad that I stuttered. It has made me stronger and I really believe that I am a better and more accomplished person because of it. But now, it has served its purpose, and I would like to experience the joy and freedom of consistently fluent speech. I am more convinced than ever that I am ready to put the pieces of the puzzle together to realize a lifelong dream. If this happens great, but if not, I'll be better than okay.

To be free from its awesome power, I must sacrifice the comfort and safety of avoidance, and embrace the embarrassment of letting go and fully showing my stuttering. The often-heard advice to "go ahead and spit it out" seems to be valid after all.

In church a couple of years ago, I was trying to think of a thought (maxim) to live by, and I came up with "Accept the moment—improve the future!" Or in other words, accept what is, and make it better. I can do that. To achieve great things, we must work hard to cross the gap between the idea and the action to make it happen. As Mahatma Gandhi said, "Satisfaction lies in the effort, not in the attainment, full effort is full victory." I have worked hard, but I will work harder and smarter to achieve full victory.

And the Steps to Victory Are...

First, look on the pursuit of fluency as an exciting challenge and enjoy the journey. A good attitude is a key to success. Second, eliminate avoidance and seek out situations that offer challenges. Third, monitor. Fourth, open up and stutter smoothly and easily and forward. Fifth, incorporate the concept of "Today for Tomorrow." Stuttering is a disorder of great complexity and diversity, and to escape its control, I must pay the price today. I must build for the future. By desensitizing my fear, I will have less anxiety and be able to speak better. And sixth, accept being a stutterer. When these six steps become second nature to me, I will catch the tiger.

And the Winner Is (or Will Be) Me!

Author: Larry R. Padgett.
Larry, born in Glennville, Georgia, has been at the West Virginia Network in Morgantown, West Virginia, since 1969. He and his wife, Linda, have been married for thirty-eight years and are the parents of one son and two daughters and the grandparents of eleven. Larry is the author of two books, the co-author of an additional two, and has published numerous scientific articles. He is especially pleased with his key role in creating the West Virginia statewide tele-communication network, which he named the West Virginia State Unified Network (WVSUN), and in his design and trademark of the WVSUN logo.

414-001-TR-ST-001-2001

"I Decided Then and There to Become a Speech Therapist…"

A BIRTHDAY CARD ON THE DOOR OF MY CLUTTERED OFFICE quotes a member of the National Stuttering Project: "When people ask me if I have stuttered all my life, I always tell them, 'Not yet.'"

I grew up on a cattle and sheep ranch in the Rocky Mountains of northwestern Colorado about fifty miles north of Steamboat Springs with my parents, brother, and sister. Looking back, my family, relatives, and neighbors valued hard work, directness, honesty, and a sense of humor. And my mother, especially, placed a high premium on getting a good education. We were isolated: Our closest neighbors were a half-mile away. It was a 20-mile drive to a one-room store and 70 miles or nearly two hours to a town of 1500 with "real" stores. I was the only one in my grade, and for most of the five years, all of the other four to seven students were first cousins, and my Aunt Grace was the teacher.

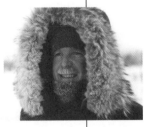

Ken on a dog-sledding trip near Fairbanks, Alaska, in 1990.

I have stuttered ever since I can remember. My mother said that my brother, who is fifteen months older than I, "stuttered," and I imitated everything he said and did. He quit, and I didn't. Years later as a client during high school, I did ask my parents if there were any other relatives who stuttered, and was told there was no one else. No one, that is, until 1988 when I was talking with my dad a few years before his death. He remarked, "Oh, I used to stutter."

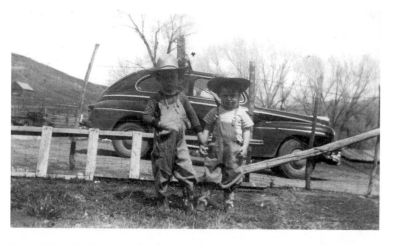

"Cowboy" Ken, on the right, holds hands with brother, David, in 1948.

Incredulously, I asked, "Why didn't you ever mention that before?" "You never asked," was his answer. Dad was a rancher; he was always wonderfully supportive of everything I tried to do but never completely understood the nuances of my speech pathology career.

There were no speech therapy services in northwestern Colorado in the late '40s and early '50s. That was true through the '60s as well. I do remember vaguely being taken to Denver as a young child and talking to a lady. This was my mother's attempt to find out at the speech therapy department at the University of Denver what might be done about my stuttering. My parents were told, "Ignore it, and it will go away." They did; it didn't. I stuttered all the way through elementary school and during junior high and high school in Steamboat Springs. And, in retrospect, I'd rate my severity level as moderate. I didn't let it hold me back academically, but I have the common painful memories of stuttering (severely in *my* mind) trying to get a date, doing oral reports, and trying to tell jokes. But I could sing fluently, and, following in my grandpa and Dad's footsteps, I often entertained people with cowboy songs.

> My parents were told, "Ignore it, and it will go away." They did; it didn't. I stuttered all the way through elementary school and during junior high and high school in Steamboat Springs.

Except for a strange two-month interlude, no one ever mentioned speech therapy to me during these years. That interlude was when I was in the sixth grade. My dad used to guide deer hunters from California, and one of the hunters was president of the school board in the little desert town of Maricopa, California. He invited me to come live with his family for a year and to see a speech therapist in their school. I went there in early October and stayed for about two months. Then, just before Christmas, I rode the train all the way back to Rawlins, Wyoming. I guess I got homesick after I got home, and, so, unfortunately, I did not return. The interesting thing about this period is that I saw the speech therapist only once, and I was completely fluent during the entire stay with my new family and my first experience in a "big" school. My stuttering returned during the 100-mile car trip from Rawlins to our ranch in Colorado.

After two and a half years of high school, I asked my mother about trying to get some help. That led to my first therapy, an eight-week summer program in Laramie at the University of Wyoming Speech Clinic.

After two and a half years of high school, I asked my mother about trying to get some help. That led to my first therapy, an eight-week summer program in Laramie at the University of Wyoming Speech Clinic. I had lots of individual and group therapy experiences. But what I remember is that a therapist taught me some techniques called cancellation and pull-out, and for the first time, I felt like I had some control. I had something to do when I felt paralyzed by the stuttering. By the end of the program, I was completely fluent in all situations. I decided then and there to become a speech therapist and to solve the problem of stuttering. That was just before my senior year of high school.

I gradually relapsed, but I was undaunted about my career decision. I entered the speech pathology program at Colorado State University as a student and also began receiving individual therapy in the speech clinic there. I had a new graduate student clinician every quarter and attended a once-a-week stuttering group therapy session run by Bill Leith. Everybody used an approach developed by the late Charles Van Riper, no doubt the world's leading authority on stuttering. There was lots of emphasis on developing a "thicker skin" or desensitization. Towards that end, once I was taken by my female student clinician and her assistant into a woman's shop, and told to ask the clerk, "Does a woman wear the same size padded bra as regular bra?" while voluntarily faking my most severe stuttering. The clerk promptly called the police thinking that I was trying to distract her while the women shoplifted.

I also had lots of outside practice using the voluntary control techniques of cancellations and pull-outs. Overall, I did very well but just could not seem to maintain my gains with any solid consistency outside the therapy situation. In retrospect, I was, in some ways, the perfect client for students, because I always showed up and tried hard. At the same time, I probably enjoyed the attention of my attractive female student clinicians too much and, perhaps for that reason, was not particularly motivated to get finished.

All that changed about the first of April of my sophomore year. Bill Leith, who was chair of the department, called me in with my new graduate clinician (a quiet, no-nonsense kind of person). He instructed her as follows, "Every time Ken reverts to his real stuttering, just grab his arm and jerk him out of the situation." Moreover, he not-too-subtly indicated to me that if I did not get control of my stuttering in the ensuing quarter, I might find myself out of the program.

This hit me like a thunderbolt, but I didn't know why at the time. Almost overnight, I felt under control almost all the time, and, in fact, often felt like I had no stuttering at all. But the interesting thing is that whenever I faked my old stuttering or just thought about being a stutterer, I would instantaneously go back to the old feeling and occurrence of stuttering. I discovered that I could play either role—the fluent speaker or the stutterer—whenever I wanted. More important to me at the time was the incredible amount of free-floating anxiety I was experiencing. I literally felt like I could jump out of my skin. It was two weeks—a period that seemed like two months—before I could get an appointment to talk with Bill. Funny. I don't remember what was said when I finally did talk to him, but something settled in my mind and emotions. That was my major therapeutic turning point.

I always had a strong desire to experience another culture. And, being an idealist in those days, after my bachelor's degree, I joined the Peace Corps and began training to go to Turkey. We studied Turkish 6 to 8 hours a day, and I was fluent (that is, with little or no stuttering) during the first several weeks. Then, as I became more skilled (or more "fluent" from a language-learning perspective), stuttering began to plague me again. This continued for the next two years. I was pretty good at foreign language learning, especially the sounds of the language, and became quite

> In retrospect, I was, in some ways, the perfect client for students, because I always showed up and tried hard. At the same time, I probably enjoyed the attention of my attractive female student clinicians too much and, perhaps for that reason, was not particularly motivated to get finished.

proficient in Turkish. But I stuttered nearly all the time. The better I got, the more I wanted to speak as a native, and the more likely I was to stutter. But, like my early years, I never let it hold me back; I went ahead with conversations, and occasionally, was quite fluent. In the rare instance that my listener didn't notice that I didn't look much like a Turk, I could sometimes even pass for a native speaker. When I returned to the US and stopped speaking Turkish, I returned to my relatively fluent English-speaking self and have remained so for thirty years.

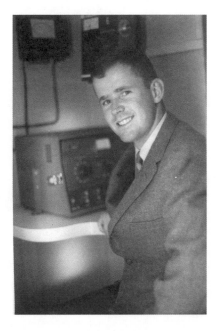

Ken St. Louis poses with equipment on a mobile research van in 1968.

Stuttering is not even among my top ten problems now. For the most part, I don't stutter very much or at least very significantly. Often, I have absolutely no difficulty. And, unlike most of the other stutterers I have known, I generally don't have to concentrate on my speech at all. But, I still don't like making telephone calls, especially to people who may not be interested in talking to me. Occasionally, I get caught in a "doozie" of a stutter (for me) in such situations. And I did relapse to some extent a few years ago, due in part to the stress of standing in front of a camera while teaching a course on satellite and in part to dealing with my mother's debilitating emphysema and death. Another situation that generally evokes obvious stuttering—and almost always to my surprise—is when I talk to my siblings or cousins. Generally, when I find myself stuttering more than usual, I do some voluntary stuttering (Yes—stuttering on purpose!) on some words or in some situations that I would just as soon not say or enter. That seems to reduce the tendency to avoid or struggle and get me back on track.

A big part of my story as a stutterer is that I want to help others who stutter. I have discovered that one of the ways I can be most helpful is through my research activities. Unfortunately,

Ken and Princess at home in West Virginia.

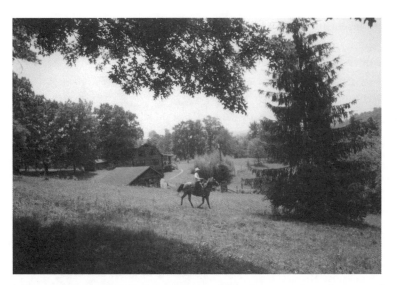

however, there is very little money available for research in the area of stuttering, although public education, clinical treatment, and self-help advocacy seem to do well. Nevertheless, my dream is to create and contribute my time and talent to an international stuttering research institute that will address problems in stuttering which can only be answered by collaborative, international research. I now know that I won't solve the problem of stuttering, but for my remaining productive years, I would like to leave an active research institute as my legacy.

...my dream is to create and contribute my time and talent to an international stuttering research institute...

Author: Kenneth O. St. Louis.

Ken is the editor and major contributor to this book. He holds advanced degrees in speech-language pathology and has devoted his professional life to learning and sharing as much as he can about the problem of stuttering. Though they often seem remote to his daily work routine as a university professor, clinical supervisor, and researcher, he has never lost his love and respect for the outdoors, rural living, and the wonders of nature.

415-001-TR-ST-001-2001

The Journey
from a Coal Town

When I was young, I used to think about what kind of profession I could pursue, who I could marry, and who my friends could be. The visions of my daydreams were similar to those filling many other children's minds. I often thought it would be fantastic to hear my voice—vibrant and smooth—come from a radio in my living room. I thought it would be wonderful to have this kind of choice, to be able to stand up and say what I wanted to say and not think or worry about the upcoming words or sounds that might cause me to block.

I used to envy the children around me who could choose radio careers. The same children viewed talking much like breathing— they didn't think about it, they just did it. People like me who stutter do not have that privilege. Not only do I think about talking, I agonize over the words that I can-

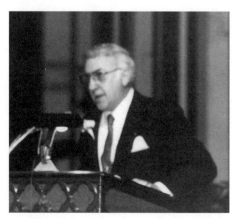

Sidney Lee delivering the commencement address to University High's class of 1986. He was completely fluent.

not say and continually try to think of words that I can substitute to continue speaking freely. This continual "find and replace"

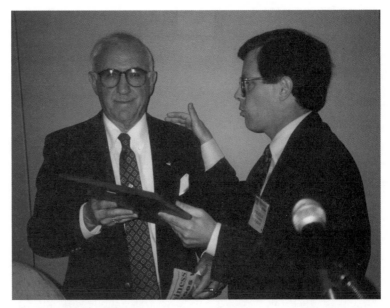

Sidney Lee receiving the Pearl S. Buck Award in 1995 from David McQuain. The West Virginia Education Association presents just one award each year to a non-educator who has made outstanding strides for education as well as the community.

technique requires a great deal of agility, a characteristic necessary for stutterers to accomplish a task that "normal people" easily take for granted.

I fittingly chose a career as an accountant. When you're an accountant, you sit at a desk, you aren't meeting the people, and you don't have to sell yourself. While career searching, I knew that many would possess the same qualifications that I did, but they would have one tremendous advantage—they could speak fluently. Therefore, I have pushed myself to work harder, be more conscientious of the things that I do, and try hard to know as much as possible about the subject at hand.

> This continual "find and replace" technique requires a great deal of agility, a characteristic necessary for stutterers to accomplish a task that "normal people" easily take for granted.

For example, as an accountant, a lot of people come to me and expect to receive the best service possible in exchange for their payment. Because many people view stuttering as a handicap and view the person that stutters as having a mental deficiency, I have to prove myself knowledgeable enough for the client to return.

Aside from work, I often must work a little harder to prepare myself for responsibilities within the community. I am often asked to present speeches such as keynote addresses for community audiences of over one thousand people. Two speeches that I have given stand out most, one for an Honor Boy/Honor Girl nomination and one for a University High School 1986 commencement address. Because I stutter, I must prepare considerably to know enough information about the subject so that I feel in control of the group. Therefore, I research, research, and research again.

I think stutterers have a sensitivity about themselves that makes them want to work a little harder, dig a little deeper, and do a little better job than the average person. Maybe we feel that we have to prove to the world that we are normal and that we are okay, or at times, better than okay.

> Maybe we feel that we have to prove to the world that we are normal and that we are okay, or at times, better than okay.

One traumatic childhood event greatly inspired me to accomplish things above and beyond necessary limits. During grade school and the Great Depression, I experienced what I like to refer to as "the word that lasted forever." One of my classmates, a boy rather large for his age, much bigger than I, and probably older, began one of my days of second grade on a sour note. With his broad shoulders head-on and his square scowling face he called me "a dirty Jew" on the way to school. I actually performed a quick check on my hands, face, and clothes, looking for visual filth, but I was no different from the other kids.

After the name-calling incident with this classmate, I sat in reading class with an already lowered self-esteem. We had just finished a passage about rabbits finding water in the early morning during the time of a drought. The teacher asked where the rabbits could possibly find water during a time when none was to be found. Every other child in the class stared back at her in silence while my hand flew into the air eager to answer.

"Dew" was the answer. I tried to tell her. I tried to prove to that bully that although I may belong to a different religion than he, I knew the answer that dumbfounded him and the rest of the class. "D-D-D," I could only say that letter over and over from my pursed lips. Children laughed. I tried with all that I had, but I could only look at my teacher with pleading eyes to communicate my answer. She did not come to my

> "Dew" was the answer. I tried to tell her. I tried to prove to that bully that although I may belong to a different religion than he, I knew the answer that dumbfounded him and the rest of the class. "D-D-D," I could only say that letter over and over from my pursed lips.

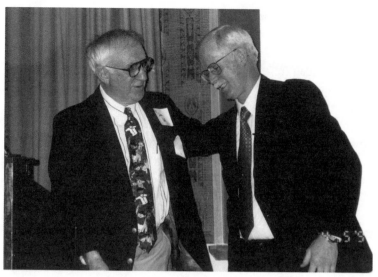

Sidney, on the left, introducing Ken St. Louis. In 1999, Ken invited Sidney, a fellow stutterer, to introduce him when he received a Benedum Scholar Award.

rescue. That day will never be forgotten. To my knowledge, up to that point I didn't stutter.

For a long time after that day, the people I communicated with had the opportunity to see and react to all of my facial tension, eye blinking, straining, neck vein protrusions, and prolonged vocal sounds. That day was the beginning of my life-long journey to try and reach a fluent stage. In whatever I do or did, it became very important to me that I did not stutter.

I feel that I have accomplished so much in my life. I had to really try hard to achieve this fluent stage in life I now enjoy and that I longed for. I put forth an effort that the average person doesn't consider. I can now stand in front of the public much like I dreamed of many years ago as a child and give a speech and receive a standing ovation. My self-esteem rises and my self-confidence skyrockets each time I stand in the doorway after a public speech and receive handshakes from the members of the audience for a job well done.

In my opinion, in every stutterer's life there is a defining moment—a magnificent moment—when one suddenly discovers he or she has broken the chain of disfluency! For me, that happened on May 31, 1986. The main auditorium of the West Virginia University's Creative Arts Center was filled to capacity, and I was about to deliver the commencement address to the University High School class of 1986. I can't describe it, but a calm spread over me and I just knew, without a shadow of a doubt, that I would be fluent. The standing ovation after the talk told me so; it happened and I call it a miracle! Since then, without hesitation, without reservation, I've spoken at many important functions without blocking.

Successes like these build on one another much like a pyramid of confidence. They have made me realize that although I may be a minority as a stutterer in the world of fluent speakers, it doesn't matter. We all have problems, imperfections. The schoolboy who looked down on me for my religion and for having a speech problem had one thing in common with me that day. Although he felt in some ways that he was better than I, I noticed that not only did one of my shoes have a hole in the rubber sole with cardboard peeking through, but so did one of his. (I might explain that during the Depression, when holes appeared in the soles of one's shoes, it was common practice to insert cardboard to keep out the mud and snow.)

I know now that it doesn't matter where you are from or where you start from, it is where you are going that counts.

My self-esteem rises and my self-confidence skyrockets each time I stand in the doorway after a public speech and receive hand-shakes from the members of the audience for a job well done.

Author: Sidney Donald Lee.
Sidney is the proud father of four children, each the bearer of a master's degree. Sidney has been a long-time supporter of his beloved alma mater University High School (UHS). He helped start the UHS Foundation and has been very involved in their scholarship program. The UHS library, which now bears his name, has especially ben-efited from Sidney's vision and generosity. In 1991 he wrote his autobiography, "...and the Trees Cried," which has enjoyed multiple print-ings. At the age of seventy-nine, Sidney enjoys taking university classes, piano lessons, and volunteering.

416-001-TR-ST-001-2001

The Gift
My Stuttering
Gave to Me

I THINK THAT I HAVE STUTTERED FOR AS LONG AS I HAVE TALKED, but it had no effect on my life until my transition from high school to college. Up until that time, I could give speeches, I could head church services, and I could talk to large classes. I was never embarrassed that I stuttered. If someone made fun of me, I would probably laugh at him or her.

Meg celebrates both her master's degree and her reconciliation with stuttering.

While preparing for graduation from high school and going to college, something snapped inside of me and I became very self-conscious of my speech. I began developing ideas about getting out on my own, becoming my own person, and beginning my own life. I did not see stuttering as an adult characteristic and I wanted to rid myself of it, or hide it at all costs. From that day on, I could not have been chained and dragged to speak in front of a group. Despite the preacher's request, I wouldn't lead church service. I also developed what I call "phone phobia." I would not talk on the phone; I hated it! I became very afraid to call people. I'd sit beside the phone at eighteen years of age, my hand clutching the hideous object, and cry.

At this time I decided to begin speech therapy at the college clinic. Prior to this therapy, I had received therapy from the school speech-language pathologist from second until tenth grade, with extra sessions from an outside therapist. I didn't benefit greatly from those services. In my opinion, I was not emotionally ready for therapy. But, by the time I enrolled in therapy at the college clinic, I was ready to conquer my problem and was more motivated for therapy.

> I'd sit beside the phone at eighteen years of age, my hand clutching the hideous object, and cry.

Throughout high school, stuttering was "just another problem" to be dealt with like every other problem in my life. I always handled them on my own and accepted help from no one. I would work through it alone, get it done, and I would be fine. Once I'd made up my mind to "tackle" my stuttering, I tried to follow my familiar problem-solving pattern. With stuttering, though, you can't really do that unless you know how to control it, and I didn't know how. I felt that I had let myself down. My self-esteem dropped and I felt that I couldn't accomplish the goals that meant the most to me, such as getting accepted into physical therapy school. An interview loomed at the end of the application process. I felt I could not get over that hurdle because I stutter worse around people I don't know and in high-stress situations. Getting accepted seemed out of my reach.

> Once I'd made up my mind to "tackle" my stuttering, I tried to follow my familiar problem-solving pattern. With stuttering, though, you can't really do that unless you know how to control it, and I didn't know how.

My friends at the time always tried to help me in any way they could. For example, my boyfriend loved to problem-solve, and he thought that by forcing me to face my fears, my stuttering would be cured. He was aware of my fear of the telephone and would make me call when we wanted to order a pizza or get the movie listings. Although his attempts were well-intentioned, they never helped me. My anxiety just worsened.

My friends would also try to raise my self-esteem and keep others, who were not aware of my problem, from hurting my feelings. They became very defensive. For example, I was introduced to one of my friend's male friends. I was talking to him and stuttered. The guy I'd just met almost said

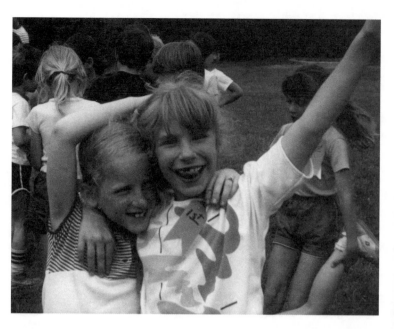

Meg on the right, age seven, at Field Day celebrating first place with friend Missy, before Meg named her stuttering a "problem."

something to me about it, but before his mouth could form the words, my friend smacked him really hard and told him, "Shut up, she stutters."

My close friends have always accepted my problem. In fact, most of them say that if I didn't stutter, I wouldn't be Meg. Other friends or acquaintances with whom I come in contact, however, are not quite as accepting. For example, a classmate that I occasionally talked to would make a comment about my stuttering each time I talked to her. She would say something like, "Having a hard time aren't ya, can you speak or what?" I still remember her comments to this day. It came to the point that I just avoided her. I didn't want to explain my speech difference to her. I didn't think much of her and I didn't wish to bring attention to my speech or myself.

Another example that stands out in my mind involved this guy that I know from my home town. He and I stood in adjacent lines at the bookstore at the beginning of the semester. He said hello, I spoke back, and we began to talk about our majors. He asked my major, and because I always have a problem saying physical therapy, I stuttered. He started laughing and said, "Well, it's obvious that you're not going into speech pathology." I was

> She would say something like, "Having a hard time aren't ya, can you speak or what?" I still remember her comments to this day. It came to the point that I just avoided her. I didn't want to explain my speech difference to her.

infuriated. For the first time I stood up for myself and let him know that I didn't appreciate his comment. He apologized, and I walked away feeling better about myself because I stood up for who I was.

Reactions such as these, and having this stuttering problem, have changed my viewpoints on humankind in interesting ways. I have developed sympathy for people with problems, indifferent to the type of problem they battle. The smallest things that everyone seems to take for granted, such as easily saying words, are very important to people for whom it doesn't come easy or may be impossible. I think that some people who know that I stutter think, "Meg stutters, no big deal." But it is a big deal. It's a huge deal for me, and learning to control it is an even larger issue in my life.

I remember the day I was moving out of my house and an old friend whom I had not seen in a while stopped by. I started talking with her and she stopped me mid-conversation and said seven beautiful words: "I thought that you used to stutter." My eyes probably gleamed with joy that day, because I knew that therapy was improving my control of my stuttering enough so that an old friend could notice a significant difference.

I had accomplished enough to be happy with myself. I was satisfied and could openly admit that I was comfortable with being a stutterer for the rest of my life. I have trained myself to be less than excellent. I realized that no one can be perfect. Stuttering has taught me that I can be okay in life without being perfect. I have a stuttering problem, but I can be as good as I can be and like myself for it. I think this is something that everyone needs to learn and living with stuttering has given me that opportunity.

Author: Meg Coleman Carpenter.
Meg is currently a physical therapist in her hometown of Princeton, West Virginia. She is a stepmother of one daughter. Aside from providing physical therapy for others, Meg enjoys weight lifting, playing the piano, and reading.

417-001-TR-ST-001-2001

I was infuriated. For the first time I stood up for myself and let him know that I didn't appreciate his comment. He apologized and I walked away feeling better about myself because I stood up for who I was.

I Chose to Swim

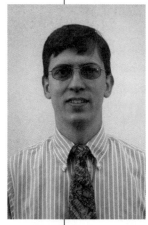

Jay Hanna today.

CONVERSATION ALWAYS PRESENTED A PROBLEM FOR ME. It was difficult to get into and participate in a conversation because my stuttering occurred more often at the beginning of a sentence. I couldn't spit out the first word. I would rehearse the first two or three sentences in my brain before I said anything.

I would take as long as thirty seconds before I could join in. My need for a pause prohibited me from getting a word in edgewise in normal conversation. You just can't pause for that amount of time in impromptu conversation. After I did get started, people could not understand me and often stopped paying attention to what I was saying because the words seemed to rush out, and I slurred them all together.

My self-confidence suffered for the longest time because I felt like all the other kids were talking and having fun while I couldn't jump into the conversation. My quietness made me appear shy and further hurt my self-image. I sometimes poked fun at myself because of my stuttering. I would try to begin a sentence and jumble up the words or start stuttering. I would whack myself and say, "Spit it out, Jay," to make the person that I was talking to feel less pressured and awkward about the stuttering.

Stuttering really didn't seem like a big deal to me until high school. I started getting into situations in which I needed to speak

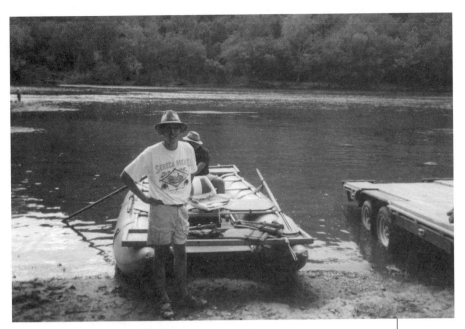

Here's Jay choosing to float. He already knows how to swim!

in front of different civic and school organizations. However, I feared trying to speak in front of a group and beginning to stutter. This fear made my stuttering worse.

At this time, I decided to bite the bullet and start speaking in front of people despite my fear. I accepted a few opportunities where I had to speak in front of people at school functions. I encouraged myself to concentrate really hard and after I got through the first couple of minutes of a public speech, it became really easy. The more I spoke, the more confidence I gained. The more confidence that I gained, the more the problem started to go away.

I feel like I overcame the problem because of my determination. I approached my stuttering the way I learned to swim. I used to be scared to death of water. One day, I just jumped into the deep side of a lake and decided that I was going to sink or swim. I was embarrassed that I couldn't swim just as I was embarrassed that I couldn't speak in front of a group. So, instead of drowning, I just swam to the other

> At this time, I decided to bite the bullet and start speaking in front of people despite my fear. I accepted a few opportunities where I had to speak in front of people at school functions. I encouraged myself to concentrate really hard and after I got through the first couple of minutes of a public speech, it became really easy.

shore. Stuttering was the same way. I just decided that I was going to start speaking in front of a group of people and either sink or swim.

Because I was so afraid of speaking in front of people and so self-conscious of my stuttering, I forced myself at an early age to start speaking publicly. I began much earlier than a lot of other high school kids. While colleagues still spoke of their nervousness when speaking in front of groups, by the time I entered my professional life, public speeches never really bothered me. By gathering the determination to jump into the deep end and practice the feared unknown, I gained the confidence to overcome my stuttering both physically and emotionally.

> I approached my stuttering the way I learned to swim. I used to be scared to death of water. One day, I just jumped into the deep side of a lake and decided that I was going to sink or swim.

Author: Joseph (Jay) L. Hanna.

Jay is a husband of sixteen years and a father of two girls. He is currently an engineer in Morgantown, West Virginia, and was originally from Keyser, West Virginia. At the age of thirty-six, Jay enjoys hunting, fishing, and all outdoor activities.

418-001-TR-ST-001-2001

A Day in the Life
of a Stutterer:
Trauma in the Drive-Thru

L IKE THOUSANDS OF OTHER COLLEGE STUDENTS, ON MOST days I have to grab a quick lunch between classes. Traffic is too bad to travel back to my apartment, and thirty minutes doesn't allow time to make anything anyway, so I choose my lunch from one of the many fast food destinations near campus.

I remember one of these lunchtime incidents clearly. I pulled into the parking lot at McDonald's and searched for a spot. I caught a glimpse of the line inside; people were impatiently lined up from the counter to the trash cans at each register. Glancing at my watch, I realized that I didn't have time to park, wait in line, and arrive at my gym class on time.

Unfortunately, I retreated to the drive-thru. I probably would have risked the embarrassment of being late for class and waited inside if I could have found a parking place. Instead, I steered my car between the curbs lining the drive-thru and prepared to order. There were no cars in front of me, and I felt myself becoming nervous as I inched toward the order screen. "Welcome to McDonald's, may I take your order?" Her words seemed to bounce at me like a snarling dog. I had to think quickly. I would have really liked to order the chef's salad. I knew that I couldn't get

Jennifer dressed, not as a clown, but as high school valedictorian.

that out. If I ordered the chef's salad, I would then have to tell her the type of dressing and order a separate drink. No way. I could have quickly written my order down. I can always say things smoothly when I have them written down; "I'm ready to take your order. May I help you with something?" Her words again startled me, bringing me back to reality. I didn't have time to write it down. I could have sung my order into the speaker. Wouldn't the crew at McDonald's have had something to laugh about all day if I had sung, "I'd like a chef's sa-l-l-l-l-l-l-lad with blu-u-u-u-u-u-ue cheese," into the speaker? Well, that was out of the question. I had to settle for a number five with Sprite, which was much easier to say.

As my heart rate slowed to normal, I pulled around to the window. "That will be $5.09." She didn't look quite as much like a snarling dog as she sounded like one coming through the speaker. I wished that I could have ordered inside. I could have stalled the cashier by studying the menu board a little longer, until I was ready to state my order. The drive-thru cashier could not see my face; therefore, I had to speak on impulse, which was impossible for me to do without stuttering.

> Wouldn't the crew at McDonald's have had something to laugh about all day if I had sung, "I'd like a chef's sa-l-l-l-l-l-l-lad with blu-u-u-u-u-u-ue cheese," into the speaker? Well, that was out of the question.

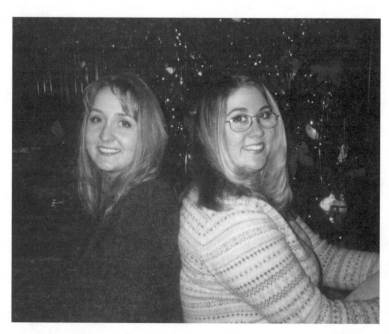

Jennifer, on the right, enjoys the company of her sister Jody on New Year's Eve, 1999.

As I took my brown paper bag of greasy fare, I mumbled, "Thanks," and sped away to my gym class a little late. It was paradoxical that I punished myself by taking a gym class, yet, on the way ate a chicken sandwich and fries. That day, I remember wishing that my parents and sister were still with me everywhere that I went. They used to order for me so that I got what I wanted when I wanted it, despite the situation. I would have liked a chef's salad that day, but sometimes I make sacrifices to save myself from embarrassment because of my stuttering.

After eating my sandwich in four bites and sitting through three red lights, I made it to my gym class a little late. I quickly shut my car door and ran to meet my classmates who were already walking around the track. As I joined their steps in unison, one of them said that she thought she knew my roommate and asked me who I lived with. I tried to answer her, but no sound left my lips. I looked away, as if trying to think of her name, and prepared myself to form the words. I then said her name. My classmate asked, "Did your mind go blank or what?" I jokingly replied, "Yeah, it's been one of those days." I just let them think that I couldn't remember her name.

I stuttered while asking for her daughter one time in high school over the telephone. Her mother asked me why I was so nervous and I didn't know how to answer her. Therefore, I tried to avoid calling her, always hoping she would call me instead.

I finished the gym class still scolding myself for seeming absentminded in front of my classmates. As I got into my car to drive home, I thanked God that the day was almost over.

Driving home, I began thinking about looking for a part-time job. I was limited in places of employment because of the speaking requirements of certain jobs. Most of the jobs available were cashier jobs at fast food restaurants. I couldn't work at one of them because I was afraid I couldn't ask someone what he or she wanted in the drive-thru line. I couldn't work at a place and answer telephones. That ruled out a nice desk position. I'd probably look for a job where I wouldn't have to speak much; grunt work was more up my alley or something where I could work face to face with people.

I pulled into the parking lot at my apartment complex, parked the car, and went inside. Replaying the messages, I discovered that my best friend from back home had called. She seemed irritated that I hadn't called her in a while. I didn't call her as much as I used to in fear that her mother would answer the phone. I stuttered while asking for her daughter one time in high school over

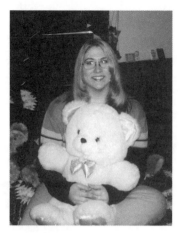

the telephone. Her mother asked me why I was so nervous and I didn't know how to answer her. Therefore, I tried to avoid calling her, always hoping she would call me instead. That evening, though, I really wanted to return her call and talk to her about jobs that she'd think I would be good at.

She would probably jokingly recommend that I become a professional clown. She knew I never stuttered in a clown suit. Despite the blue curly hair, red nose, and baggy polka-dot pants, my voice always remained smooth and free flowing while in the clown troupe in our high school. I could perform in front of small or large groups, use my high-pitched clown voice, become another person for a few hours, and speak with ease. That type of job wasn't practical in college since a circus wasn't coming to town any time soon.

I sat the phone back down on the receiver and decided to call her later. She knew me; I hoped that she would call back instead. I had had a rough day and wasn't ready to deal with talking on the telephone.

Jennifer and Snuggles at home in North Spring.

Author: Jennifer Lee Davis.

Jennifer is a junior in biology at Concord College in Athens, West Virginia. She is originally from North Spring, West Virginia, and is the younger of two daughters. Jennifer is twenty-one years old and enjoys singing both alone and with a choir, playing tennis, and collecting stuffed animals.

419-001-TR-ST-001-2001

Secrets within Us

Stuttering has always been a very prominent and personal aspect of my life, a communicatory handicap which I repressed for years. I was, in effect, a "closet stutterer," refusing to acknowledge my problem with my family and friends. Like any young person I was unwilling to accept any impediment that made me different than anyone else. Mercifully, my marred speech eventually straightened through my own intense practice. Once I felt comfortable speaking I did so carefully, making silly public excuses for my occasional lapses. It wasn't until near the end of my undergraduate career that I finally accepted my flaws, during an internship where I met someone who had not had my luck correcting her own stuttering problem.

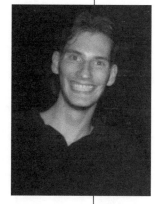

Patrick Niner.

"So, have you ever had s-s-speech therapy?" Leaning over my shoulder, Katrina's eyes never wavered from my computer screen.

Surprised, I opened my mouth, then closed it again in a ridiculous fashion. *Great,* I thought, annoyed. When had I done it? Must have been when I said "Internet." Or maybe "site," words that started with "s" were always trouble.

I'd been researching ways to publicize the company via the World Wide Web, and been in a hurry to give Katrina a report before the other interns and I headed out to lunch. I wondered how much of it she had heard before my lapse. She looked at the screen with feigned interest, but when she glanced back at me I could tell she wasn't as indifferent as she seemed. There was curiosity in her face, and even a bit of nervousness.

When I first met Katrina two months before, it took no time to notice that her speech was tarnished by an obvious stutter. I'd made note of it, but as we worked on different floors of the building, I'd never had the chance to study it further. I'd never intended to tell her that I also sounded like a skipping record on occasion, "b's" and "c's" and "s's" rolling around in my mouth just waiting for my breath to spit them out and move on to the next sound. I'd watched her at a comfortable distance, but never made it a point to actually talk to her. This project, though, had brought us together, and in less than a day she'd exposed me.

I realized I couldn't escape, or use the typical excuses like fatigue or anger or inebriation as I normally would, so I kept it simple. "Yes, I had therapy when I was in grade school. So, do you see how if we submit our URL to this address the engine will review our site and…"

"You're a s-s-stutterer?" Katrina's lips turned up a bit and she turned to face me. I recognized her expression, the same one I'd seen when she'd met our newest intern, an African-American student from across town. She was pleased, happy to meet someone like her.

"No, not really," I answered, keeping my voice even and carefully pronouncing each word. "Occasionally, but not often. It happened all the time when I was a kid, though." Uncomfortable with where the discussion was heading, I made it a point not to look at Katrina and turned away slightly.

"No kidding?" Katrina pulled up a chair and straddled it. I checked the computer's clock. Time for lunch.

"Did you get help after that?"

"N-n-not after fifth grade." My heart jumped.

"Why not?"

I gave up pretending to study the computer screen and swiveled my own chair around to face her. "It wasn't helping, not the way I wanted it to. See…" I watched Katrina as I spoke, and

> When I first met Katrina two months before, it took no time to notice that her speech was tarnished by an obvious stutter. I'd made note of it, but as we worked on different floors of the building, I'd never had the chance to study it further.

decided if she were interested, I might as well tell her. Over about four minutes, I gave her a short account of my speech history, how I initially couldn't pronounce the "r" sound, and how I'd entered the school's speech therapy program in third grade to correct it. Later the therapist and I worked on stuttering, but I soon tired of being pulled from Reading, my favorite class, to go to the weekly hour sessions. I didn't mention how I eventually refused to do the exercises and clammed up whenever the therapist asked me a question, or how I folded my arms during our last meeting and, in classically conformist fifth-grader style, flatly denied I was any different from my classmates. Katrina listened attentively, asked a couple questions, then smiled and released me for lunch, making me promise to talk to her before the day was out.

When I returned, I found a flier on my desk advertising the local university's group therapy program. "We meet tonight," Katrina told me later. "The m-m-meeting starts at seven-thirty. You s-s-speak well; maybe you can tell us your story and give us some tips?"

I drove home that afternoon and wondered what I was going to tell them. Would they ask me what I did to not stutter? Easy, substitute words on-the-fly for others I have problems with. Stop talking when I feel myself choking up and pretend I can't think of the right word. Or, best of all, blush like a fool and comment that I really had too much to drink last night.

Maybe it was curiosity, maybe it was a desire to get out of my sweatbox apartment and into the air-conditioning of a school building. Whatever it was, as I sweated in the night's July heat I decided to go. As I walked outside I passed my landlady, who inquired where I was off to during such a hot night.

"A meeting," I said. "A stuttering support group."

"Are you running it?" she asked.

"No, no, I'm participating."

"You stutter?"

"No, not really."

At the university I found myself sitting in a blissfully cool conference room, next to a grinning Katrina who said she was happy to see me. There was a dark-haired, youngish-looking man in a business suit a few seats down who pleasantly introduced himself as Milton, and a silent fortysomething skinny guy across the table who wore red spandex pants and a sweatshirt.

When the therapist and his assistants arrived, they greeted the group. I noted that the assistants, probably graduate students, led the meeting instead of the therapist. After a few minutes of small talk, one assistant asked what "targets" we would be working on tonight. I was confused, and watched as Milton rose from his chair. He brushed away a bit of lint from his jacket sleeve.

> I noted that the assistants, probably graduate students, led the meeting instead of the therapist. After a few minutes of small talk, one assistant asked what "targets" we would be working on tonight.

"Hello. My n-n-name is Milton…" he began.

And I'm an alcoholic, I finished mentally, pleased at my originality.

"…and tonight I will work on t-t-taking a full breath of air, and t-t-try easy onset for my 'c' words." He exhaled, everyone nodded encouragingly and he sat.

The spandex-wearer stood (*ouch,* I thought), and introduced himself as David. According to him, he'd also try to regulate breathing, and he'd use a lot of "s" words for practice. Katrina then declared her own goals, her speech stopped many times by blocks. She didn't try and change what she was saying, though, she struggled through the words until what she wanted to say was said. I made a mental note to suggest it to her later. The silence between words when she spoke disturbed me.

I passed on the exercise, deciding that my prepared, humorous answer of "I'll try not to stutter" wouldn't be warmly accepted. Then the assistants asked that we freely answer a question.

"If there were a pill to make you stop stuttering, a medical miracle, would you take it?"

"In a s-s-second," Milton chimed in. The group tittered.

"Without a doubt," Katrina added.

"Sure," I agreed.

David sat thoughtfully. "W-w-would it have side effects?" he asked. I almost rolled my eyes. *That's a dumb question.*

"That's a good question," the assistant answered. She traded looks with the therapist, and I realized we'd played right into their hands. "If there were a side effect, like tremors or cold chills, would you take it?"

I thought about that, and I was still thinking about it as everyone else nodded away around me.

"How about hearing loss?" The grad student surveyed us. "Or nearsightedness?"

Milton pursed his lips. "I don't know about the s-s-sight thing," he said softly. "But I'd give up some hearing if I didn't have to stutter anymore."

"Me t-t-too," David said. I couldn't believe it. The assistant spoke again.

"How about if it put you in a wheelchair? Would you give up use of your legs if it meant you could speak?"

"W-w-wait a second," I spoke up, aware that I just stammered but, for once, I didn't care. "That's ridiculous. Sight, hearing, mobility; those make you f-f-far more d-d-d…"

My breath caught in my throat. I couldn't say it. I looked at the ceiling and racked my brain to think of another word, but couldn't. Everyone looked at me and I felt more pressured. The air simply wouldn't flow, and when it did a steady stream of "d's" came out.

A hand touched my shoulder. Katrina's. I looked at her, and the other stutterers who just sat and patiently looked at me, as if we were having an informal coffee break. There were no inquisitive looks or uncomfortable silences from them, things that happened so often when I'd blocked in front of friends or coworkers.

I exhaled, and repeated my sentence. "Those make you far more *dependent* on others. S-s-stutterers can rely on themselves for help."

Everyone smiled.

My breath caught in my throat. I couldn't say it. I looked at the ceiling and racked my brain to think of another word, but couldn't. Everyone looked at me and I felt more pressured. The air simply wouldn't flow, and when it did a steady stream of "d's" came out.

🌱

I attended the group for the rest of the summer, and learned more and more about the others. David had been a talented mathematics student, but had secluded himself from others because of his impediment. I imagined him alone, silently working with his numbers, fitting them into equations and making them line up perfectly, working with material that always changed but allowed no margin for error. Then there was Katrina and I, writers who loved creating symmetrical, flowing sentences that concisely told the stories we wanted, how we wanted. Perhaps bravest of all was Milton, who worked as a construction-equipment salesman and spent half his day in corporate meetings, the other half on his cell phone with clients. Despite his constant stuttering, he never quieted during the day while the rest of us sat silently behind computers.

Afterward, when I told a few friends that I was thinking of starting my own stuttering support group, they expressed surprise. "You stutter?" they asked.

"Yes," I answered. "I do."

Author: Patrick T. Niner.

Pat is a twenty-two-year-old graduate student at the University of Cincinnati. He received his bachelor of arts in English from West Virginia University.

420-001-TR-ST-001-2001

No More Constant Dread

IT WAS BEFORE A BIG GAME AND PEOPLE WERE GATHERED ON THE West Virginia University campus for the dedication of the mountaineer statue by our governor. I wanted to get up close to see a famous orator, someone who could really speak publicly. I wanted to see how he spoke, if he had a degree of nervousness. I wanted to read his face.

I discovered something that day that gave me the confidence to change my life. The speaker had his hands behind his back, and I just kind of slipped around to look at his hands. His hands were quivering. I could not believe that he was nervous and twitchy because his voice was totally controlled, unwavering. There wasn't a hint of dryness in his voice, no shakiness. His presence was relaxed, controlled, and confident, even though perhaps inside, his belly was jumping up and down. That observation has always stuck with me. It convinced me that I could control my voice. I figured if he could do it, so could I.

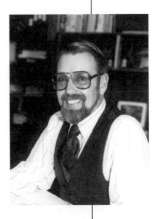

This photo of the adult Lynn Caseman shows him as the smiling and confident man he had become.

I was a graduate student at the time and had suffered with stuttering all my life. I had encountered many devastating situations, which created a need for the self-confidence that would allow me to take charge of my dysfluency. I was always on the lookout for ways to improve my speech, to boost my confidence. As a kid I used to think I was cursed by God and that I had done something I wasn't aware of, and this was my punishment.

Growing up, I had many difficulties socially. I'd call a girl up for a date, and she would ask, "Who is this?" I couldn't say my name and she would just hang up. Any kind of social interaction was hard. The stutterer lives in total apprehension all the time. People who don't stutter just take talking for granted. I developed some very negative feelings about the future. I really couldn't imagine going through life, I saw no hope. In high school, my experiences with a speech therapist who stuttered worse than I, and my observations of adults older than I with ongoing dysfluencies, contributed to these negative feelings.

> Growing up, socially, I had many difficulties. I'd call a girl up for a date and she would ask, "Who is this?" I couldn't say my name and she would just hang up.

I was definitely treated differently by others because I stuttered. In high school, my senior year in English, the teacher would not call on me, so I wouldn't have to answer. In the US Navy, it was sheer torture at boot camp. Every time we did anything, they took roll. They had two ways of identifying you or making you respond: you could yell your last name, or you could yell a number that had been assigned to you. My number was fifty-seven; I'll never forget. Of course I had problems with my name, but to make matters worse, "f" was a sound I couldn't say. I got a lot of flak at boot camp.

> My number was fifty-seven; I'll never forget. Of course I had problems with my name, but to make matters worse, "f" was a sound I couldn't say. I got a lot of flak at boot camp.

College was also troublesome. There was a guy at the time working on his doctorate in education, while also teaching at West Liberty State College. After three or four months, he called me into his office. He knew I was in education, and he told me, "Get out of education. You are a stutterer, you will never make a good educator. You will be an embarrassment in the classroom, so get out of education."

Like many stutterers, I imagine, I was interested in theories about stuttering and about different approaches to treatment. At one point in college, I heard a learning theory about synapses growing together. I realized if that's true, I could do something about my speech. From that point on, I approached my stuttering positively. I was committed to teaching myself to speak. I purposely put myself in situations where I had to say my name, where I had to say words and phrases that I could never say, for example, ordering "chocolate ice cream." I conscientiously told myself that I would restructure my synapses.

I never gave up hope. Experiences such as watching the governor speak and hearing the theory of the synapses helped me develop greater control of my dysfluencies. Now I am a completely fluent adult. Those social situations where I lived in constant dread, I don't have that now.

Author: Lynn F. Caseman.
Lynn Caseman, a resident of Middlebourne, West Virginia, is a retired elementary school principal with over thirty years' experience. He has been married to his wife, Milli, for thirty-nine years. He has three daughters: Lisa, a principal in West Virginia; Eva, a school nurse supervisor in Kentucky; and Kelli, a writer in North Carolina. He is the proud grandfather of three grandchildren, Hannah, Millie, and Jarric. Lynn was born in Wheeling, West Virginia, grew up in Wellsburg, West Virginia, and graduated from Bethany College and West Virginia University. He is currently on the faculty at West Liberty State College as supervisor of student teachers, and is also a preacher for the Brownsville Church of Christ in Brownsville, Ohio.

421-001-TR-ST-001-2001

Graduate Orals Proved
to Be My Testing Ground

I LEFT MY COMFORTABLE, FAMILIAR TOWN IN NEW HAMPSHIRE TO pursue a degree in Animal Science at Virginia Tech. I was then "dumped" into a whole new world of experiences, having left a small group of close friends behind. Then, I accepted a graduate position in reproductive physiology at West Virginia University, which introduced new people, new pressures, and a lot of oral presentations. My challenge began.

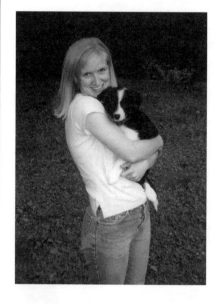

Beth and Clover enjoy each other's company. No talking necessary!

I hated public speaking. I remember sitting around a table with my colleagues the first year. Although the meetings were informal, my stomach would tighten in knots as the opportunity to present my research approached—quicker and quicker. I knew no one my first year in graduate school. Speaking seems to become easier the longer I know the people with whom I am speaking, so there was some relief. But speaking in groups remained a problem.

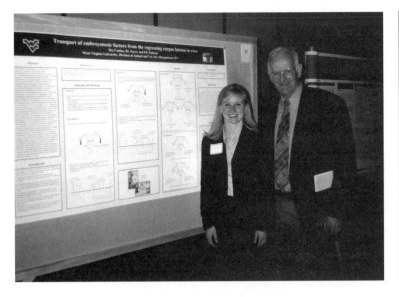

Student Beth and advisor Dr. Inskeep in front of the poster presenting Beth's graduate research.

I began speech therapy in elementary school with a very positive experience, which gave me the initiative to continue. This first therapist was very helpful, but moved out of town. I was then assigned a new therapist who misdiagnosed my stuttering as an articulation disorder. Until then, I had enjoyed therapy, but at this time I stopped attending. During high school, I was relatively fluent and did not need therapy. A small, comfortable group of friends surrounded me and diminished the need. I was also involved in various clubs and organizations and made oral speeches and won state contests, so I don't think my stuttering really ever inhibited me until later in graduate school.

My therapist and I worked on fluency shaping through easy onset and controlling my breathing. I found this type of therapy very helpful, but our time was limited to thirty minutes per week.

I moved to Virginia for college, with a whole new group of friends. By my junior year I again sought out a therapist. This time it was at a clinic in Roanoke. My therapist and I worked on fluency shaping through easy onset and controlling my breathing. I found this type of therapy very helpful, but our time was limited to thirty minutes per week. I became frustrated because I could not carry over the techniques from the therapy room into daily conversation.

In my first oral presentation in graduate school, I was required to present an hour-long speech to an audience that I felt knew more on the subject of my discussion than I did. My

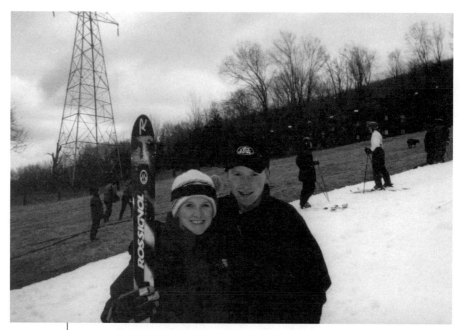

Beth and her brother Tim enjoying themselves at Beth's ski race.

experience was horrible. For the first time in my life I wanted to flee from the room and not finish the presentation. Rehashing the experience days later, I decided to inquire about the speech clinic on campus.

I consider myself to have a mostly outgoing personality, which was great for when I worked as a salesperson at Sears and World of Science. Occasionally, I would have problems with my speech. Customers would ask me, "Are you okay, is everything okay?" as I struggled through a block. Sometimes customers would engage in a guessing game with me to fill in the words that I could not say. It was irritating because it wasn't that I couldn't think of the word, I just couldn't say it. Most of the time, I ignored their attempts to help me, but now and then I would prolong my stutter on purpose.

> It was irritating because it wasn't that I couldn't think of the word, I just couldn't say it. Most of the time, I ignored their attempts to help me, but occasionally I would prolong my stutter on purpose.

I hold no embarrassment about my stuttering because it is obvious to others that I stutter and I know that I stutter. So, I do not mind discussing my problem with others. In my opinion, one of the hardest parts is when I speak fluently. I have always stuttered, and changing the way I speak is something that I didn't think about when I began to speak fluently. I realized for the first time that I don't talk the same; it feels different, rather odd.

For two years now I have been working with my current therapist on learning the techniques of cancellation, pull-out, and preparatory sets. I have also learned to stutter voluntarily when I am having a difficult day to reduce my tendency to struggle. I am reaching my goal of "stuttering well"—without the secondary behaviors, tensions, and blocks. I would not have progressed as far as I have without therapy. I have periods of very good fluency, the best was in the fall of 2000 when I defended my master's thesis. It was excellent.

Author: Beth Alyson Costine.
Beth is a twenty-four-year-old doctoral student in reproductive physiology at West Virginia University from Chester, New Hampshire. She enjoys hiking, skiing, mountain biking, and camping. Beth is thankful for the people in her life who did not allow her stuttering to slow her down and instead encouraged her to become involved in things that required speaking and interacting with people at many levels.

422-001-TR-ST-001-2001

Practice Makes Perfect

TODAY AS A TEACHER AND BASKETBALL COACH, I VERY RARELY stutter except during basketball season. I guess there's still something about the excitement of the game that just makes my speech worse. Also, the phone is still hard.

The first time that I remember stuttering was in the fifth or sixth grade when I had to read. Kids would laugh at me, especially when I answered questions in class and stuttered. I often stuttered on words that started with an "a." So, I started my sentences with "the" or something else. If I came across an "a," "an," or "and," I would put "the" in front of it, "the an," to cover it up. I stopped answering questions while knowing the answers. Instead of making As, Bs, and Cs, I could have made straight As if only I had been able to talk. It really embarrassed me. I stopped participating in school.

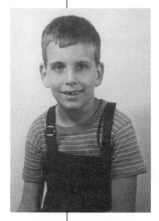

Frank in the early grades, when he still participated fully in school.

One exception was basketball. I played and was really affected by my stuttering during basketball season. During the excitement of playing, my talking was terrible. I couldn't say anything without stuttering.

Even in college, I was still shy because of the stuttering. I still wouldn't answer questions, because I didn't want people to laugh at me. As before, I knew the answers. They would laugh at you in college. When I was taking Physical Science, a professor asked me a question, and I started stuttering. I couldn't get the answer out and he just hollered at me, "Shut up!" He told me to shut up, slow down, count to ten, and start all over. Then, in the same tone, he told me that he used to be a stutterer and to go into the woods and talk to the trees.

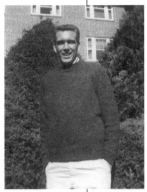

The author in 1959, crew neck and crew cut.

I went all through college stuttering. I passed, but I could have made As instead of the lower grades I got. My junior year I was able to give speeches if I had papers or an outline in front of me. But, if I was put on the spot, for example when asked a question, I could feel my whole body get nervous.

My stuttering also affected my career later in life. I didn't get a coaching job that I had wanted one year in the school system. A friend of mine knew someone on the school board. He said that one of the reasons mentioned why I didn't get the coaching job was because I would never be able to answer a question. Of course, that hurt me.

In growing up, my parents never acted like I was doing anything out of the normal. This was probably best because doing otherwise would have drawn attention to my stuttering, which would have made it worse or made me feel worse about it. They never really talked about it. My mother always approached life as, "This is where I am today. This is the way things are. Go on." That is the way she handled things and she helped me do the same a lot.

I think, without knowing it, my mother may have contributed to my stuttering. Some papers that I read on stuttering suggested that forcing a child to be right-handed when he or she is left-handed would cause stuttering. When I was born, my mother tried to get me to be right-handed even though I favored my left. But, I don't know whether this made a difference.

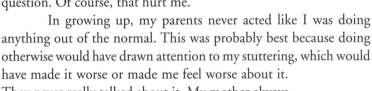

I still wouldn't answer questions, because I didn't want people to laugh at me. As before, I did know the answers.

When we first met, my wife looked beyond my stuttering. She said that she thought I was the best looking thing that she had ever seen, so she didn't care that I stuttered. She looked past my imperfections, saying that she was attracted to my disposition and laid-back attitude.

My wife has little tolerance for people who are insensitive to stutterers out of ignorance. I recall once when we were talking with another couple. The man, in his fifties or older, said, "I got so tickled when Frank started stuttering." He said that he thought it was so funny and my wife gave him a look that caused dead silence among us. He and his wife knew that he had said something stupid.

I have developed my own tactics and used some of the suggestions of others to get where I am today with my stuttering. For example, I took my professor's advice. When he suggested that I go talk to the trees, I did. It helped. I slowed down sometimes.

I also used to count to ten when talking on the phone to control my stuttering. When someone answered, I would count real slow before saying anything. I would also do that before answering questions.

I overcame stuttering on my own. In my forties, I was asked to be the lay leader for my church district, which was a huge honor. I had to speak and teach people, and that did wonders for me. It was a form of therapy for me. The more I talked, the better my speech was. I think that working as a district lay leader, going to different places, and making speeches in front of a lot of people made my stuttering go away.

I have also helped myself by reaching out to others and being more open about my stuttering. I teach, and the first day of school I ask the students to tell me their names. This year as part of

> I have also helped myself by reaching out to others and being more open about my stuttering. I teach, and the first day of school I ask the students to tell me their names. This year as part of that, I decided to tell the students that I stuttered.

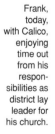

Frank, today, with Calico, enjoying time out from his responsibilities as district lay leader for his church.

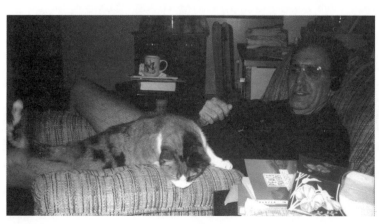

that, I decided to tell the students that I stuttered. Even though I rarely stutter when teaching, I explained that I had stuttered a lot, back when I was in school. I got them thinking about how everyone has some kind of handicap, whether it is being scared to speak up, stuttering, or whatever. I think it shocked them. It was just total silence. I went on to mention the country singer Mel Tillis, a stutterer, and how well he had done.

> I had to speak and teach people and that did wonders for me. It was a form of therapy for me. The more I talked, the better my speech was.

I have gained much from my experiences stuttering. It has made me realize that sometimes in people's lives, there are problems. I understand people who are ashamed or scared to say something because they think they are from the wrong side of the tracks, that they are different. I have a special feeling for those people because I've been there too. I've seen the looks on their faces and I know the feelings they have in their bodies when they can't answer questions. I relate to them and use this understanding as a teacher.

Author: Frank Harrison, Jr.

Frank, now age sixty, is a father of one son and one daughter and a grandfather to one grandson, Seth, and one granddaughter, Kelsey. He enjoys taking part in raising his grandchildren and in playing golf. Frank was born in Montcalm, West Virginia, and currently lives in Mullens, West Virginia.

423-001-TR-ST-001-2001

With God
All Things Are Possible

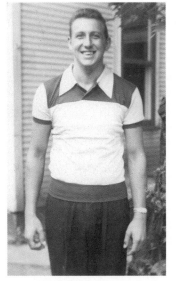

Henry at graduation from high school. He had already decided to become a minister.

Y EARS BACK, I WAS A MODERATE TO SEVERE STUTTERER. BUT, IT has been thirty-seven years now that I've been speaking fluently. As a young man, I had goals in life that I knew would be impeded by my stuttering if I did not learn to overcome it. I felt that to control it I needed to better understand the cause. Now, like most people who stutter, I could sing and not have any trouble at all. This assured me because I knew if I could sing that there wasn't anything wrong with the way that I produced my words. So, I knew that it was something else and as I reflected upon it, I determined that rejection was at the root of my stuttering.

Feelings of rejection began as early as the first grade. I did feel acceptance at home, but school was another story. I had a teacher who was very strong in discipline. She didn't just dish it out to the trouble-makers. Rather, she "rode herd" on everyone. I hope there aren't any more of those teachers around. One of the things she would do was to make us sit in a circle of red chairs to read. We would go around the circle and when it came to our turn to read, if we missed a word, we would have to hold our hands out and she would smack them with a ruler. That went on for quite a while. My feelings of self worth plunged as a young, sensitive six year old. I felt that she may have meant well, but used pretty nasty methods to get there.

I began having trouble with different words and syllables. But, I sort of came out of it after moving on to other teachers and becoming an avid reader in the fifth or sixth grade. If the teacher asked for volunteers to read aloud in the class, my hand went up. Called upon, I did pretty good.

> We would go around the circle and when it came to our turn to read, if we missed a word, we would have to hold our hands out and she would smack them with a ruler.

In my sophomore year in high school, my mother died. When that happened, my world caved in, and I really became unsure of myself, which threw me back into stuttering. I had also lost my father to death when I was seven, and recall the grief of filling out various required forms those early years. I was always sensitive about the fact that in the square where I was to write my dad's name, I had to write, "dead" or "deceased." That made me feel inferior to others and took a toll on my self-esteem. With the loss of my mother too, I lost a lot of my self-confidence.

My stuttering became more severe my senior year in high school. One memorable incident was in my senior English class when we were required to write an essay discussing what we wanted to do in life. My essay talked about how I wanted to be a minister, a decision I'd made my sophomore year. The day came for us to turn in that assignment and the teacher said, "You know, I think that it would be really nice if everyone would get up and read their paper in front of the class." And so, I thought, "*Oh horror!*" I got up when my turn came and I got through it, but I stuttered an awful lot. When I was finished, the teacher called me over to her desk and said, "Henry, you have great aspirations, but you had better change your goal. You'll never make a good minister because you can't talk."

I decided that I *was* going into the ministry. I went to Kentucky Christian College in Grayson, Kentucky, and began to work on my stuttering immediately. I had problems with anything that began with an

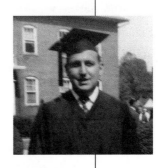

Graduation from Kentucky Christian College, where he began to work on his stuttering.

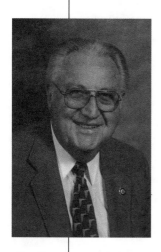

Rev. Henry B. Pratt. With God's help, he became a minister after all.

"s"—words like "six," "seven," or "sixties." If I was speaking in public and there was a word with a syllable that had an "s" in it, I knew I would just stammer and stutter until I got it out. This was always on my mind. There were some very frustrating times in my life when stuttering just overwhelmed me because I felt like I wasn't getting any place.

There were several things that helped me overcome my stuttering. For one, I realized that I could move beyond my earlier feelings of rejection and insecurity. Also, my ability to sing reminded me that I could indeed produce words and not stutter. In the end, though, the way I overcame my stuttering was that I believed I could overcome it. I looked to the Lord for help and prayed about it a lot. The more my faith in God increased, the better I did. With positive reinforcement that I could do this, I began to work by myself, in private. When I was alone I would talk aloud and read out loud. The more I read out loud, the more confident I became. I never saw a speech pathologist, but had a speech professor at college who worked with me a little bit and did encourage me to keep trying and get by myself and speak out loud. Mostly, however, it was on my own.

When I tell people today that I used to stutter, they just look at me and they have a hard time believing that was the case. As a minister, I have preached over 5,000 sermons. In graduate school, I took courses in radio and television. During the forty-plus years that I have been in the ministry, I have done a lot of television programs. Today, I am a producer of a television program that is in its fortieth year of running. I've been involved with that program for over eighteen years. I do weddings and funerals, and I don't have any problems. I feel a lot of fulfillment because at one time there were so many things I couldn't do—or thought I couldn't do. I really try to do my best and try to help others.

I never saw a speech pathologist, but had a speech professor at college who worked with me a little bit and did encourage me to keep trying and get by myself and speak out loud. Mostly, however, it was on my own.

Overcoming stuttering was something that I could not have done if I had not embraced the promise of the Lord. Those who do not have faith in the Lord would say, "Well, he just built up his self-confidence." But, to build your self-confidence, you have to have something to build it in. You have to have an object for that and my object is God. Early in life I claimed Philippians 4:13, "I can do all things through Christ who strengthens me," and God has enabled me to speak fluently.

Author: Henry Brooks Pratt.

Henry was born in Colliers, West Virginia, is married and the father of two and the grandfather of three. He has lived in Quincy, Illinois, for twenty-two years. Eighteen years ago he was the founding pastor of Faith Christian Church there, and has been active in evangelism, music, and television ministry for more than twenty years.

424-001-TR-ST-001-2001

My Struggle
with a "Demon"

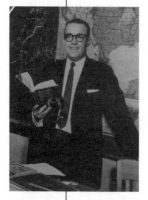

JB in 1962 at the head of a fifth-grade class in Turkeyfoot Valley Area School District in Somerset County, Pennsylvania.

Before I could overcome my stuttering problem, I had to convince myself that there was nothing wrong with me physically affecting my ability to speak. Many stutterers don't come to that conclusion. I realized I could sing and speak fine when alone. I could also salute the flag and speak in unison with a group and never have a problem. I only had a problem when I had to speak on my own. I deduced that there was nothing wrong with my voice box. Early on I decided that it must be in my head.

I went to a one-room school and began to stutter in the fourth or fifth grade. Stuttering was a great disadvantage during my school years. For example, my grade school teacher required us to memorize one poem or passage a year, like *Et Cetera, The Village Blacksmith, The Gettysburg Address,* or *Barefoot Boy.* We had to learn so many stanzas a week and stand up and recite them. Some weeks I begged off, even if I knew the piece, because I couldn't recite it. I also went all the way through high school knowing answers frequently in class, but when called upon I didn't answer because I didn't want other people knowing that I couldn't say the answer.

I would open my mouth and nothing would come out. I didn't repeat things. I would just open my mouth and nothing would come out, just like a blockage. I felt embarrassed. I was reluctant to speak out.

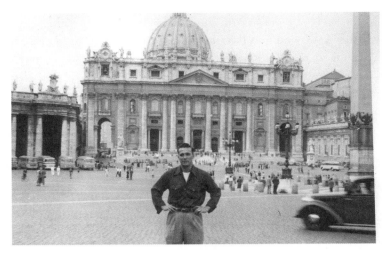

St. Peter's Square, Rome, in 1955 before college and while in military service.

Maybe my guidance counselor knew what I thought I had kept hidden from everyone because she suggested that I get a job using my hands. So, I did; I became a crane operator. This was a problem. I took a job perfect for a stutterer, but I was not satisfied. I didn't deal with anyone except truck drivers and people who pushed cars in and out from under my crane.

I read a lot on stuttering in the fifties. I know that breathing is an important part. I think in speech therapy they teach you to breathe. Free-flowing speech will follow if you learn to breathe evenly, to take your time.

I was drafted. I had a lot of time on my hands while in the service, so I would go down to the service club where they had a nice library. I got as many books as I could find with speeches from people like Daniel Webster, Henry Clay, and Thomas Jefferson. I would take them back to my room and read them to the four walls with little or no difficulty. I feel that at that time I was trying to further prove to myself that there was nothing wrong with me physically.

I was in the service two years. After being discharged, I decided to go to college on the "GI bill." I was a poor mountain boy, who shouldn't have been applying for college at that time. Most of the people I went to high school with did not go on. I was the

> I got as many books as I could find with speeches from people like Daniel Webster, Henry Clay, and Thomas Jefferson. I would take them back to my room and read them to the four walls with little or no difficulty.

exception. Plus, there was my stuttering problem. I really didn't know whether I was going to be able to make it through college or not. With that in mind, I figured if I was going to college, I might as well study something I liked. I chose history. I entered nearby California State Teacher's College in 1955

While working on my degree there, in my thirties, I came to the helpful conclusion that no one has completely fluent speech.

because it was relatively cheap with in-state tuition. Also, being concerned about making it, going somewhere close to home made sense. And so, I studied to become a history teacher. If I had known that I was going to be able to overcome stuttering completely, I might have taken a completely different course. My tenure at California State Teacher's College was happy and what many would consider most successful. I was very active in school politics, serving as class president and president of the student body. I also worked as head waiter in the school dining room.

I graduated from California and then went on to West Virginia University to get my master's, still stuttering. While working on my degree there, in my thirties, I came to the helpful conclusion that no one has completely fluent speech. I thought that many stutterers probably have their speech problem because they are striving for perfection. Every time stutterers come to what might be considered a normal pause in their speech, they see it as a problem. I learned that I could stop for a second or two and look for the word or even go right on after being stuck for a second.

With this acceptance and understanding of my stuttering, I took my first teaching job, still stuttering, but with strategies for hiding it. Because of my stuttering, I developed a unique teaching method that seemed to work well for both me and the students. I didn't lecture. I talked very little. Some people would say that's a good way to teach because it means the students have more opportunities to speak up and participate. I would write questions on the board and call on someone to read those questions aloud.

I never went into a meeting cold—I had to have some idea of what I was going to say.

I would then point out the page in the book that the answers were on and facilitate student discussion.

After receiving my bachelor's and master's in secondary education and teaching for a while, I went back to school to receive my elementary certification. I went on to teach fifth grade, sixth grade,

and then to become a school administrator who directed the activities of fifty
or sixty people a day. I often spoke at
assemblies of three to four hundred
people. I also held faculty meetings
and worked with large groups of people
and parents and had no particular
problems at all. I probably prepared
more than any other school administrator. I never went into a meeting cold—
I had to have some idea of what I was
going to say. Then, and to this day,
probably few are aware of the fact that I
have had this speech problem. Still, I occasionally come to words I
can't say, but because of my education, my vocabulary is large enough
to choose a different word. I've noticed "m's" and "l's" for some
reason are hard to say.

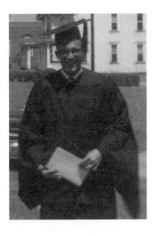

1959,
graduating
from
California
State
Teacher's
College of
Pennsylvania.

I believe I overcame stuttering by realizing that I did not
have to speak perfectly. Most stutterers are striving for perfection
and do not realize that very few people have free-flowing speech.
All people pause and stop and say, "uh," and other things in the
process of speaking. Pauses are not a cause for alarm; most listeners
do not even notice them. When I learned to accept my pauses, much
of my anxiety went away and with time, my speech became more
free-flowing and fluent.

Author: Jackson B. (JB) Thomas.
*JB, age sixty-seven, is a retired public school
teacher and administrator originally from
Markleysburg, Pennsylvania. He is the husband
to Judy, father of two, and grandfather of two.
He lives in Uniontown, Pennsylvania, and
enjoys collecting coins and political items. JB
refers to his stuttering as the "demon" that
pushed him into college, graduate school, and
leadership positions. But maybe, he comments,
he may have just had to prove that he could.*

425-001-TR-ST-001-2001

CHAPTER 3

Stuttering 101: Some Basics

What is stuttering?

We're not really sure...

It is probably not necessary to define stuttering for those of you who have experienced it. You know what it is and what it feels like. But, for those of you who don't stutter, although you generally recognize stuttering when you see and hear it, the mystery of the problem begs for a precise definition. Unfortunately, this is not as easy as it may seem; clinicians and scientists have been trying for most of recorded history to define stuttering. Have we progressed beyond the "pick your favorite definition of stuttering" stage? Yes, but not as far as we would like to be. We now know that stuttering is more than Wendell Johnson's tongue-in-cheek summary: "Stuttering is what the stutterer does not to stutter." We also know that it is less than Jon Eisenson's description as a "transient disturbance in communicative propositional language." Charles Van Riper's definition, "stuttering occurs when the forward flow of speech is interrupted by a motorically disrupted sound, syllable, or word or by the speaker's reactions thereto," still holds a lot of appeal.

> "People just don't know what the problem is or how to fix it. It could be a neuron that doesn't arc electricity between two places. It does in your brain, but it doesn't in mine 99.8 percent of the time." —*m, age 43*

But we have achieved some success.

To deal with this lack of consensus, a group of speech-language pathologists who have special interest and expertise in stuttering identified four different definitions of stuttering. Two of the definitions referred primarily to the outward symptoms of stuttering such as repeating, prolonging, or otherwise struggling to say words or parts of words. Two others included definitions that refer to the cause of stuttering, such as neurological or coordination problems affecting speech, or to a feeling of being out of control. I recently contributed a definition to a book for people who stutter which pulls together most of those elements. Here it is:

"Stuttering results from involuntary neuromotor breakdowns affecting the coordination of respiration, phonation, and articulation of speech. It typically—though not always—is 1) experienced by the speaker as a loss of voluntary control in saying words; 2) manifested as excessive and/or abnormal sound/syllable repetitions, prolongations, audible or silent blocks, or attempts to avoid these behaviors; and 3) associated with or triggered by variable amounts of psychic stress and negative emotion." (St. Louis, K. O. (1997). What is stuttering: Some more current additions. In S. B. Hood (Ed.), *Stuttering Words*, p. 12. Memphis, TN: Stuttering Foundation of America.)

Despite the difficulties and challenges in defining stuttering, we now consider stuttering disorders to fall under the umbrella term of "fluency disorders."

Want more information?

In 1999, the American Speech-Language-Hearing Association's Special Interest Division 4 (SID 4) on Fluency and Fluency Disorders developed official guidelines on terminology related to the field. These guidelines summarize definitions and relevant background on such terms as "stuttering," "fluency," "fluency disorder," "disfluency," "normal disfluency," etc. These are reprinted in this book in *Appendix F: Terminology Pertaining to Fluency and Fluency Disorders: Guidelines.*

Who stutters and when?

Lots of people stutter, but you may not know anyone who does.

If you are reading this book, you probably know someone who stutters (maybe several people) or you stutter yourself. But clearly, those of us who stutter are in a small minority of the general population. Many people are not aware of anyone who stutters and have never heard it—in person or even on television, in a movie, or on the radio. Let me summarize what we know about the distribution of stuttering in the population as well as some things we do not yet know for sure.

One percent stutter now and five percent stutter at some time.

The rule of thumb is that slightly less than one percent of the population stutter at any given time. A number of good research studies have shown that the 1% is fairly accurate in the US, Western Europe, and most other developed nations. This is roughly equivalent to the concept of "prevalence." But the issue is more complicated: the likelihood of stuttering is related to one's age, sex, other stutterers in the family, and possibly, certain environmental factors. This brings up the tricky concept of "incidence," or the rate of new occurrences of stuttering in previously stutter-free populations. Here the research is not as strong at this time and provides less precise estimates. The best estimates generally are in agreement and predict that about 5% of people will stutter at some time in their lives. Most stuttering begins before the first grade, usually at about three to four years of age, but can begin as early as two years or as late as adulthood. Although much that has been written about the problem focuses on stuttering in older children or adults, it is important to realize that most stutterers "outgrow" or recover completely from their problem with no outside help. Actually, about four out of five or 80% of young stutterers will recover if stuttering that lasts only a few weeks or months is included. The so-called "spontaneous recovery" rate drops to about 50% if cases in which stuttering has been present for a year or more are counted. Thus, it has been said that stuttering is a disorder of childhood. Even so, chronic (ongoing) stuttering occurs in about 20% of cases and continues into adulthood. Although rare, spontaneous recoveries do occur in adulthood. But, most of these late recovering stutterers have done so by learning how to manage their stuttering, either from speech therapy or on their own.

Boys stutter more than girls do.

That's not the whole story either. Three to four times as many males as females stutter, especially among adults.

"Mel Tillis, he's a country music singer, he's very famous. A lot of people think it is an act, but it's not. There's something you all so-called experts can study on. How can a man sing and be a country music star, very successful in life? He's had many hits, and yet when he talks, he stutters bad, real bad." —m, age 60

"It gradually went away. The only time I find myself stuttering is if I get real excited about something. That's about it." —m, age 59

In the disorder of stuttering—and lots of other conditions such as reading problems—boys are definitely not the stronger sex. At every age, there are probably more boys than girls stuttering. However, the difference is not so great during the three-to-four-year-old period, pointing to the trend that young girls are more likely to recover from stuttering than boys.

"I've read reports that say it is inherited. There were six of us kids, three of us stuttered, three of us didn't. I don't know, but how come if it's inherited, how come I and my two brothers stuttered, and a brother and two sisters didn't stutter? I mean, it doesn't make sense." —*m, age 60*

Stuttering often runs in families—but not always.

We also must factor in a genetic component. We know for a fact that stuttering runs in families more than it does not, yet the genetic determinants are complex. Although some excellent research is currently underway, we cannot predict exactly who will stutter and who will not. Even so, if one or both parents stutter, their child has a considerably greater chance of stuttering than if neither of them stutters or used to stutter. The genetic influence seems to be more potent if the mother stutters. How can this be? Remember two facts: more boys than girls stutter, but girls are more likely to recover. Well, if a girl does not recover and continues stuttering into womanhood, it is likely that she has more of whatever genetic influence that fosters stuttering than a boy who continues his stuttering into manhood. Having said this, it is worth emphasizing that these are no more than statistical probabilities. Many people who stutter have no known relatives who stutter, and many, many people who never stuttered come from families where stuttering is common.

Want more information?

Ehud Yairi, Nicoline Ambrose, and others at the University of Illinois have published a series of studies on a longitudinal study of children who stutter. Their work is very important in understanding the risk of developing stuttering, onsets, recoveries, and the early nature of the problem. The following article provides a succinct review of the critical literature as well as a somewhat controversial point of view about how long to wait to treat a young stutterer. Other researchers are not sure we should wait to treat preschool stutterers.

Curlee, R. F. & Yairi, E. (1997). Early intervention with early childhood stuttering: A critical examination of the data. *American Journal of Speech-Language Pathology, 6*, pp. 8-18.

Saskia Kloth, Floor Kraimaat, and Peggy Janssen in Utrecht, The Netherlands, have also carried out a highly significant longitudinal study that tells us a great deal about the risk of stuttering and the factors that predict recovery.

Kloth, S., Janssen, P., Kraimaat, F., & Brutten, G. J. (1998). Child and mother variables in the development of stuttering among high-risk children: A longitudinal study. *Journal of Fluency Disorders, 23*, pp. 217-230.

Stuttering is often not the only communication problem.

Stuttering is often not the only speech or language problem a person has. As many as 40-50% of those who stutter have other problems such as articulation disorders (that is, an inability to say certain sounds such as "s" or "r" correctly), language problems (for example, various difficulties understanding or using words, grammar, or meaning), or voice problems (for example, hoarseness). These problems are often overshadowed by the stuttering and, therefore, may not be particularly noticeable.

"Cluttering" is another fairly rare fluency disorder that often occurs along with stuttering, although it can also occur alone. This disorder has been described for more than a hundred years, but compared to stuttering we know very little about it. Authorities don't completely agree on how cluttering should be defined, but there seems to be growing consensus that clutterers talk too fast and have jerky, irregular speech. These speech rate problems contribute to other difficulties that include, for example, too many of the normal disfluencies such as fillers and revising words, leaving out sounds or syllables in rapidly produced words or phrases, or being particularly difficult to understand.

"I'm not saying what I want to say quick enough. And when I try to say it at the speed my brain is going, then it becomes a stuttering process. It's really confusing for people to understand sometimes what I'm saying, especially if I get nervous." —*f, age 44*

"I actually had two speech problems when I was little. I had the stuttering thing, and I couldn't enunciate my 'r' for some reason. Is that common?" —*m, age 22*

Want more information?

With my colleagues at West Virginia University, I have been involved in documenting the coexistence of stuttering and other speech and language disorders. There is an extensive review of much of this work as well as some of my own research in a monograph.

St. Louis, K. O., Ruscello, D. M., & Lundeen, C. (1992). Coexistence of communication disorders in schoolchildren. *Asha Monograph*, No. 27.

My colleague Florence Myers and I have been very much involved in researching cluttering. The following brochure and chapter summarize much of that work.

St. Louis, K. O. (1998). *Cluttering: Some Guidelines*. Memphis, TN: Stuttering Foundation of America.

St. Louis, K. O. & Myers, F. L. (1997). Management of cluttering and related fluency disorders. In R. F. Curlee and G. M. Siegel (Eds.). *Nature and Treatment of Stuttering: New Directions* (2nd Ed.). New York: Allyn & Bacon, pp. 313-332.

> "I guess it started when I was in probably the sixth grade. I noticed that I had a stuttering problem and the stuttering problem really only occurred when I was nervous, for the most part. Time went on. I had a hard time in high school because we had to get up and do speeches a little bit. I was pretty timid, I'm kind of a shy guy anyway, and so I didn't participate as much as I should have. I enjoy talking to people, but when I get around people then I would really clam up." —*m, age 35*

Stuttering is universal.

Finally, although we suspect that there are differences in the prevalence and incidence of stuttering in different countries, cultures, or races, the best available evidence suggests that stuttering is present in all human societies and has existed throughout recorded history. There is an ancient Egyptian hieroglyphic for stuttering, scholars have concluded that Moses stuttered, and words or well-known phrases for stuttering have been found in virtually all natural languages.

Stuttering changes over time; most stutterers get better with no help, but some don't.

Now, regardless of the above risk factors, let's take a look at how stuttering changes over time. As we have said, with children most stuttering gets better or goes away in four out of five cases. In the one out of five that persist, it often gets worse over time. In many cases, a young child starts stuttering with repetitions of short words or syllables like "I-I-I-I-I-I-I want a cookie" or "Pi-pi-pi-pi-pi-pick me up" with little obvious awareness of the problem at all. This progresses to beginning awareness of the difficulty and the addition of tension in the voice and sometimes comments like, "I can't talk." Later, the person who stutters often begins to discover "accessory behaviors" or tricks that help him or her get a difficult word started or completed. These take on a wide variety of forms: blinking the eyes; saying "uh" to stall or get started; forcing a word with excessive tension in the voice, mouth, or face movement; avoiding certain speaking situations; substituting synonyms for feared words; and so on. These accessory behaviors are learned very rapidly because they are usually very effective initially in allowing the speaker to go on. Unfortunately, they typically begin to lose their effectiveness over time. And, instead of abandoning them once they no longer "work," the stutterer often incorporates them into the stuttering pattern without realizing it, making the stuttering symptoms even worse and more complex.

Stuttering usually varies in some predictable ways.

For reasons that are only partly understood, the chronic stutterer tends to stutter more on initial versus later syllables in words, on stressed versus unstressed syllables, on syllables beginning with consonants versus vowels, on longer versus shorter words, and on uncommon versus common words. He or she often experiences less stuttering in the following situations: while relaxed versus excited (negative or positive), while feeling rested versus feeling fatigued, after a period of stuttering versus just starting out, during speech with friends and family versus with strangers, or during free conversational interactions versus answering specific biographical questions.

After a few years of stuttering like this, a person's self concept and self-esteem usually are affected, and he begins to think of himself as a person who is unable to talk like other people. Because of this, the stuttering begins in small or large ways to determine the person's choices, from whether to call a friend on the telephone or answer an incoming phone call, to the kinds of social relationships one enters, to what one chooses to do or study for a career.

"When you talk on the phone, you have to say who you are. You can't say, 'My name is, you know, Jane Fonda,' or anything made up like that. You have to say who you are and that's a real catcher. When you are stuck with things that are an absolute fact, that you cannot get around, and you're in one of these emotional funks, you really are caught, and you just would rather not do it. You avoid doing it at all costs because there is no substitute for your name, your address, the town you're from, when you were born, ..." —f, age 54

...But not always.

In some cases, the above sequence of changes in stuttering is very short indeed, especially in late onset stuttering. In other cases, stuttering does not develop past the early stages. This is particularly true of mild stuttering that the person is able to manage without professional help.

What happens during and because of stuttering?

Stuttering usually consists of repetitions, prolongations, and blocks.

As I mentioned, stuttering can be defined in terms of certain symptoms or behaviors that are most common in the problem. These are known as "core behaviors" and include syllable repetitions ("muh-muh-muh-muh-maybe"), prolongation ("mmmmm-mmaaaaaybe," or blocks ("[tense silence]....................maybe.") Normal speakers rarely have these core stuttering behaviors; instead, their speech often contains normal disfluencies such as fillers ("like," "well," "I mean," or "um"), short hesitations ("Can you hold this [short pause] thing for me?"), revisions ("Hand me the pli—the screwdriver), or phrase repetitions ("Jeremy likes—Jeremy likes—Jeremy likes turkey and dressing"). Repetitions of single-syllable words ("Be-be-be-be-be careful!") are sometimes normal disfluencies, but sometimes they are early symptoms of stuttering, particularly in young children.

There is much more to stuttering though—accessory behaviors that can usually be seen, and feelings that may be less apparent.

Accessory behaviors—or tricks the person who stutters adopts to help get started on a difficult word, stall or postpone saying it, get through it once it starts, or avoid it altogether—were mentioned earlier. There is a wide variety of accessory behaviors, virtually as diverse as the imaginations of those using them. It won't come as a surprise that these are a major factor in determining why stutterers stutter in so many different ways.

Feelings and thoughts about stuttering are highly significant as well. As a stutterer becomes aware that a word is not coming out in the way he somehow knows very vividly is "right," lots of troubling feelings may accompany the experience. After the initial surprise or realization about stuttering is no longer present, one of the most common feelings after struggling to say a word or sentence is embarrassment. After all, who wants to make a fool of himself? Embarrassment may later give way to fear and anxiety about stuttering or about speaking in general. As stuttering becomes a person's usual way of talking, anger, shame, and guilt may surface as well. Other feelings that often accompany stuttering are frustration at speech being so time consuming or hard or a kind of "existential frustration," asking "Why me?" or "Why can't I do something about this?"

Teasing of stutterers is common.

The experience of being teased for stuttering is extremely common. Other children—and a few adults, who don't understand why the person repeats or prolongs her sounds—often mockingly stutter themselves, give the person a name like "Stutter-box" or laugh and whisper behind her back. As innocent as these common childhood and adult interactions may seem, many stutterers are deeply hurt by them. "Sticks and stones may break my bones, but words can never hurt me" is not true for most stutterers. And yet, some people who stutter are not adversely affected; these people seem to have a special resiliency that allows them to insulate themselves from teasing or to simply laugh it off.

"The worst teasing came from my family, believe it or not. One time, during Easter—this is kind of funny—I wanted something. I really can not remember what, and a relative got fed up and finally yelled at me, 'Spit it out!' So, being young, I spit on my kitchen floor. I got completely punished for that." —m, age 39

Want more information?

Marilyn Langevin at the Institute for Stuttering Treatment and Research in Edmonton, Alberta in Canada has developed a curriculum that is widely used in Canadian schools to help teachers reduce teasing and bullying of children. Although designed for stuttering, it applies to all kinds of teasing and bullying.

Langevin, M. (1997). Peer teasing project. In E. Healey and H. F. M. Peters (Eds.), *Proceedings of the Second World Congress on Fluency Disorders.* pp. 169-171. The Netherlands: Nijmegen University Press.

Most people think stutterers are nervous and shy, even though it is not true.

Even if most people are outwardly sympathetic to stuttering—and that appears to be the case—there is a stereotype that is widely held in all societies where stuttering has been investigated. The stereotype is that stutterers are nervous, shy, fearful, quiet, and reserved. Many lay people, professional people, young people, older people, people who don't stutter, and people who stutter, hold this view. By definition, a stereotype is a perception that is not borne out by the facts. As we will see below, there is little evidence that stutterers are in fact any more nervous, shy, fearful, quiet, or reserved than nonstutterers happen to be.

Want more information?

Gordon Blood has compiled a very detailed summary of research pertaining to negative stereotypes and stigma associated with stuttering. Also, Ken St. Louis, Scott Yaruss, Bobbie Lubker, and others are conducting an ongoing series of studies designed to develop a public opinion poll that can be translated and used anywhere in the world to assess public attitudes toward stuttering.

Blood, G. (2000). *The stigma of stuttering: Centuries of negative perceptions and stereotypes*. Paper presented at the Annual Convention of the American Speech-Language-Hearing Association. Washington, DC.

St. Louis, K. O., Yaruss, J. S., Lubker, B. B., Pill, J., & Diggs, C. C. (2001). An international public opinion survey of stuttering: Pilot results. In H-G. Bosshardt, J. S. Yaruss & H. F. M. Peters (Eds.), Fluency disorders: Theory, research, treatment and self-help. *Proceedings of the Third World Congress on Fluency Disorders in Nyborg, Denmark*. International Fluency Association, pp. 581-587.

Why do people stutter and how are they different from people who don't stutter?

We are getting closer to understanding the cause of stuttering.

As a speech-language pathologist (SLP) with a specialty in stuttering, perhaps the most frequent question I am asked is "What causes stuttering?" It's a very good question, but one that has defied a solid answer since men and women first started asking it. The easy answer is, "The cause of stuttering is unknown." But, if I were to take the witness stand, even though this answer qualifies as "the truth," it is neither "the whole truth" nor "nothing but the truth." We know for certain that stuttering is not an action from a vengeful God, nor is it caused by demons, ghosts, or spirits, although a disturbing number of people still think so. We also know that far more often than not, parents or caregivers cannot identify any specific shock, trauma, or fright that can be associated with the onset of stuttering in children. In any case, whatever theory is put forth to explain the cause of stuttering, it must square with an astronomical amount of research that has been carried out with people who stutter, comparing them to those who do not.

"It seems like a Jamaican myth that I started my stuttering because when I was born my mother tickled me on the bottom of my foot." —m, age 19

Thanks to the research efforts of many in recent years, the answer to the question "What causes stuttering?" is not nearly as remote as it was a generation ago. Let me use three common causal categories—physiological, psychological, and learning—to summarize the views that appear to be most commonly agreed upon at the beginning of the 21st century.

Most likely, stuttering has a physiological cause.

More and more evidence suggests that the typical stuttering that begins in childhood and gets worse over time has a physiological basis. Physiology, of course, refers to the body and its functions. This includes the function of the brain and nervous system, where the most likely stuttering-related defects lie. Going deeper, it is likely that stuttering involves a subtle coordination control problem of the muscles of breathing, voicing (that is, making sounds), and articulating, primarily or especially during real, communicative talking. Basically, it is a problem in getting all the speech movements to occur with the correct force, in the proper sequence, at precisely the right time. At an even deeper level of explanation, it is likely that the problem in stuttering stems from an inability to make necessary changes in command programs to certain muscles in response to error messages sent to and received by the stutterer's brain. Furthermore, it is likely that many individuals who stutter are influenced, perhaps negatively, by their tendency to use unusual pathways in the brain, such as pathways in the right side rather than the left side, or by an overly active pathway that usually comes into play only during emotionally charged experiences. No doubt some of these differences are at least partly determined by the stutterer's DNA genetic blueprint that differentially affects males versus females.

It is important to note the existence of a very rare type of stuttering known as neurogenic stuttering. In these cases, stuttering begins after a clear case of brain damage. There are some marked differences between most of these cases and the common type of stuttering I have mainly described in this chapter.

> "Well, the brain says, 'Don't want to say that word.' When the brain says, 'Don't want to say that word,' you don't say that word. That's the brain for you. If he doesn't want you to say that word, you just don't say that word." —m, age 18

Want more information?

One of the best sources of information available on all aspects of stuttering is Oliver Bloodstein's *Handbook*. Bloodstein does a masterful job of summarizing the mountains of research data on physiological studies of stuttering.

Bloodstein, O. (1995). *A Handbook on Stuttering* (5th Ed.). San Diego, CA: Singular.

Nancy Helm-Estabrooks has written several chapters describing the nature and treatment of neurogenic stuttering.

Helm-Estabrooks, N. (1999). Stuttering associated with acquired neurological disorders. In R. F. Curlee (Ed.), *Stuttering and Related Disorders of Fluency* (2nd Ed.). pp. 269-288. New York: Thieme.

The jury is still out about whether or not there is one or many causes for most cases of stuttering. Certainly, there are multiple possibilities. Genetic differences are likely to be present in most cases, but in some cases there is no evidence of stuttering in one's extended family. Also, even though stuttering rarely has a documented psychological cause, there are cases where it clearly and specifically follows a psychological trauma. And, to make things more complicated, consider that even the outward manifestations of repetitions, prolongations, and blocks are not in and of themselves proof of real stuttering. It is possible for a nonstutterer to fake a stutter that is indistinguishable from real stuttering to an innocent bystander. It is also possible for stutterers to produce faked and real stuttering as well. My guess is that there are multiple causes of stuttering but that we will eventually begin to identify clusters of causes that apply to various subgroups of people who stutter.

Want more information?

Anne Smith and Ellen Kelly have written about a changing model rather than a stationary model of stuttering. In other words, they suggest that what is going on in the stutterer's brain, nerves, and muscles provides a better idea of what is going on than does whether or not the stutterer happens to manifest a repetition, prolongation, or block.

Smith, A. & Kelly, E. (1997). Stuttering: A dynamic, multifactorial model. In R. F. Curlee & G. M. Siegel (Eds.), *Nature and Treatment of Stuttering: New Directions* (2nd Ed.). pp. 204-217. Needham Heights, MA: Allyn & Bacon.

"I was involved in an automobile accident, and I noticed about two to three months had passed and I began stuttering."

—*m, age 48*

Psychological problems may be present but generally are not the cause.

Theories suggesting psychological causes of stuttering have been around since the beginning as well. Considering the common stereotypes and beliefs about stuttering mentioned earlier, it is no surprise that many people seek to explain stuttering as a psychological problem. Stuttering does get worse under stress. Its initial onset sometimes follows psychological shock or trauma, such as being bitten by a dog or a family going through a divorce (although these are not the typical patterns). The fact that most stutterers can speak with total fluency when they are singing or talking alone to themselves also reinforces the notion that it must be "all in the head."

I won't attempt to summarize the theories, but I'll mention a few. One Freudian-based theory held that the mouth movements seen in stuttering resemble the sucking and biting movements of infants. Freudian theories are not taken very seriously today, probably due to the objectionable language used to describe them, but similar views have replaced them. One theory is that stuttering is a symptom of an underlying neurosis, namely a conflict between

"I started when I was probably about five or six. My twin brother started and I used to tease him about it. Then he quit, and I started. Then it started again when I was probably seventeen or eighteen, and my brother got killed in a car wreck." —*m, age 40*

wanting and not wanting to express anger and other emotions caused by perfectionist parents.

A great deal of research using all sorts of psychological measures and tests has been carried out to determine if groups who stutter are different from those who don't. A few studies have found differences, but most investigations (and especially the studies that used better scientific procedures) have shown very few, if any, differences between the two groups. The only area in which stutterers are consistently different from nonstutterers is social adjustment.

> "Probably the reason I overcame it was my mom and dad instilled in me that it was important for me to overcome it, but not that it was anything wrong or bad or they didn't constantly pick on how I talked. They would correct me but they wouldn't dwell on it. They would give me time to talk. They would tell my sister to be quiet a little so I could talk, but it wasn't said there was anything wrong with the way I talked." —f, age 45

Another line of research carried out for more than two decades beginning in the 1930s at the University of Iowa investigated the parents of young stuttering children to see if they were maladjusted. The chief investigator, Wendell Johnson, said the answer was yes. He believed that overly critical parents labeled normal disfluency as stuttering in their children, setting into motion a vicious cycle whereby the child would try not to "stutter" (that is, not to use normal disfluencies). In so doing, the child would acquire more disfluencies because of the stress. These normal disfluencies then gradually changed into real stuttering. Johnson's interpretation of his results determined an entire generation's beliefs about the cause of stuttering. A paraphrase of his diagnosogenic theory was that "Stuttering begins in the parent's ear, not the child's mouth."

A careful reading of Johnson's data revealed that the parents were not "maladjusted." His own and subsequent data showed that parents of stutterers were not significantly different from the parents of nonstuttering children (according to the standardized psychological tests), although a few had greater expectations for when their children should reach various developmental landmarks (such as saying their first word or walking).

Johnson's theory discouraged clinicians from working with children who stutter because he advocated telling parents to ignore their children's stuttering so that it would go away. Sadly, Johnson could not have known that 80% of young stutterers would get better regardless of what was said or not said to them. He believed it was the advice he gave that caused the recoveries. Unfortunately the 20% who needed help were abandoned until much later. Ironically, we now know that the earlier stuttering is treated, the better the results.

Stuttering is typically worse under stress, and stutterers often experience fear and other negative emotions during speech. But, with the possible exception of social adjustment, stutterers are no more likely to be maladjusted than nonstutterers. How can we reconcile these opposing observations? The solution is that stuttering is likely to cause psychological problems—*not* that psychological problems cause stuttering.

Want more information?
Again, Oliver Bloodstein's book is an excellent source of results of studies of the personalities of stutterers or their parents.

Bloodstein, O. (1995). *A Handbook on Stuttering* (5th Ed.). San Diego, CA: Singular.

...But there are a few psychologically based cases of stuttering.

There probably is a small subgroup of stutterers who do have some significant psychological problems. Most clinicians have seen an occasional client for whom some of the early psychological theories seem to fit. However, these cases of so-called "psychogenic stuttering" are rare.

Learning plays a role in some behaviors and feelings but does not cause stuttering.

Is stuttering a habit that was learned? The consensus among researchers and clinicians is "no." A few models have tried to explain how someone, for example, a member of the stutterer's family, could inadvertently reward repetitions and prolongations, but these models have not been taken seriously. More relevant are theories that stuttering is "picked up" or imitated from someone else, such as a sibling or a parent who stutters. As simple as this may sound, a careful look at virtually all cases where someone has suggested that a child picked up stuttering from someone else reveals that imitation is not a significant cause. For one thing, most children begin to stutter with different symptoms (for example, whole word repetitions) from those of the other family member who stutters (for instance, a father who prolongs and blocks). Also, other children, siblings, or friends almost never begin to stutter after simply playing with a child who does.

> "Every once in a while I catch myself skipping or getting going on 'st' words for some reason. It's only 'st' words. I don't understand what it was about, but it was always that type of sound. I couldn't do it. I always had a 'st-st-st' like that on it." —m, age 21

To experts in behavior, the word "learning" has a very specific meaning related to the uses and power of negative or positive reinforcement. As I just noted, the core problems of stuttering—that is, repetitions, prolongations, and blocks—are probably not learned; however, there are two aspects of stuttering where learning seems to play important roles. Accessory behaviors, like taking a short gasp, are no doubt learned through a process of "instrumental conditioning." Here is how it works: The person is stuttering and the act of stuttering is unpleasant. If a little thing like an inhalation gasp is inserted during a stutter and is immediately followed by the ability to move ahead, the gasp is rewarded immediately and consistently by the desirable situation of being able to finish a communicative message and to get one's meaning across. At the same time, the gasp ends the unpleasant circumstance of stuttering. So the next time the person stutters, he is very likely to do what worked before.

The other area in which learning plays a role is in the generalization of feelings such as fear. This is known as "respondent" or "classical conditioning," as the famous scientist Pavlov described with his dog. Remember how Pavlov was able to get his dog to salivate (the response) after ringing a bell (conditioned stimulus) after repeatedly pairing the bell with the sight of food (unconditioned stimulus). In the same way, if a stutterer experiences anxiety (response) upon saying his name (unconditioned stimulus—"B-B-B-B-B-Bill," for example), the "b" (conditioned stimulus) is automatically paired with "Bill" and, over time, begins to elicit anxiety itself. After this happens, other "b" words such as "boy" become feared just like the name, "Bill."

How do people cope with or manage their stuttering?

People can and do manage stuttering on their own.

As strange as it seems, speech-language pathologists often either fail to recognize or forget that people have been coping with stuttering for eons with no professional help. That is still true, especially in countries around the world where very few speech-language services are available. And, interestingly, it is very much the situation in the US right now as well. As I noted in *Chapter 1: Introduction*, I have been collecting stories of people who stutter for several years. I have shared this work with my speech-language pathology friends and students who were surprised to learn how many stutterers have managed their stuttering successfully without ever consulting a speech-language pathologist.

As far as I know, there are no books available that list all of the ways that stutterers have treated themselves, but there has been a long and ongoing record of testimonials throughout the centuries of ways that stutterers have learned to deal with their problems. Some of these techniques have been suggested by family or friends of the stutterer, some have been carefully thought out and tried by stutterers, and some have been accidentally discovered.

Some people who stutter believe they have been successful in dealing with their stuttering by:

Taking your time before starting to talk.

Thinking about what you are going to say before saying it.

Slowing down your speech.

Enunciating your words clearly.

"Singing" your speech.

Practicing saying certain words, sentences, phrases, or longer pieces over and over again.

Reading aloud for a period every day.

Making a joke about your stuttering early in a conversation.

Telling a person that you stutter.

Imitating other good speakers.

Making sure you have adequate breath support for speech.

Projecting your voice.

Purposely putting yourself into difficult speaking situations in order to build up your confidence.

Simply refusing to stutter.

Refusing to let the stuttering get the best of you.

Saying, "I stutter. So what?"

Doing what you have to do in spite of stuttering.

Finding or living with someone who is understanding of the stuttering.

Saying "um" before a difficult word.

"When I was in high school is when I started to learn the fact, the key, to speech therapy for me. I had read books, you know, pamphlets, and I talked to some people, and I learned that the biggest thing was confidence. And once I learned that, I started to slowly have a handle on it. As I got older, it got better and better." —*m, age 46*

Learning to substitute synonyms for words that you think you will stutter on.

Spelling a difficult word aloud and then saying it.

Choosing jobs that don't require much talking.

Getting mad.

Doing other things that don't involve talking very well.

Sharing experiences and camaraderie with other stutterers.

Talking with pebbles or marbles in your mouth (as the ancient Greek orator Demosthenes did). (I really don't recommend this one. It could be dangerous! —*Editor*)

Stutterers, themselves, discovered some therapies.

As we shall see, many of the techniques that stutterers discovered are very similar to the therapies used by clinicians and fluency disorders specialists. A number of approaches teach the person to speak slowly in highly specific ways, and virtually all of them require some degree of learning to monitor or pay attention to speech in a new way. Most speech-language pathologists would not recommend some of these self-management techniques because they recognize that the techniques can compound the problem in other ways. For example, stutterers may feel that they are successful if they avoid speaking, but this avoidance often leads to isolation and feelings of inadequacy.

People who stutter are like people coping with any other disability. Nearly all of them have summoned some amount of courage and resourcefulness to make the best of their speech disorder. Many have so successfully managed their stuttering that they no longer believe it to be a significant issue in their lives.

"I was trying to say 'I.' They're going, 'Spell it!' How do you spell 'I?' I'm like 'Ahhhhh...' I started pointing at my eyes and they said, 'Eye?' and I said 'Yeah.' So I finally got it out." —*m, age 43*

"I know I can stand up in front of 300 people and give a speech now, no problem. Because, I don't know, I taught myself how to. The thing I think that helped me the most to overcome it was actually two little marbles. You take two of them, put those in your mouth, and it makes you speak slowly and clearly. If you don't speak slowly, you're likely to swallow them." —*m, age 24*

(Don't try this. —Editor)

The personal stories in this book have been chosen to illustrate approaches or attitudes that have been helpful. My hope is that these stories will provide insights (to stutterers and nonstutterers including speech-language pathologists) into stuttering treatment that few textbooks on the subject will include.

Formal stuttering therapies generally are combinations of a few similar techniques and approaches.

I would now like to summarize the most common ways speech-language pathologists treat stuttering in North America and Western Europe. I must be honest, however, and first point out that there are many other approaches that are used besides those I mention below. Certain approaches have been omitted because the majority of "experts" in the field do not regard them as favorably as those that are included. Other approaches may be missing simply because they have not yet been publicized or they are untested or too new to be widely recommended.

I try to keep an open mind about new and different approaches because my experience has been that there never has been one best approach to stuttering treatment. On the other hand, research has shown that there is a great deal of ignorance and fear among speech-language pathologists about treating stuttering, and the cumulative therapy experiences of those who stutter reflect that. Often the therapy suggests uncertainty or lack of current knowledge by clinicians. Summarizing the most widely accepted approaches might assist stutterers or their families in seeking treatments that stand the best chance of success.

Different experts have categorized the various approaches to stuttering therapy in useful and creative ways. The following five general approaches reflect my colleagues' categories as well as my own experiences as a stuttering client, a teacher, and a clinician: fluency shaping, stuttering modification, contingent management, linguistic hierarchy management, and desensitization/counseling.

Fluency shaping is currently the most widely used type of therapy, but it is not quite as popular as it was in the early 1990s.

Fluency shaping is a term that means different things to different experts, and as a result, a great deal of confusion exists as to which therapy techniques are fluency shaping procedures and which ones are not. I prefer to restrict the term fluency shaping to those techniques that specifically *teach* the stutterer to learn to speak in ways that are smooth, easy, and incompatible with stuttering. In other words, if you learn to talk this certain new way, you can't stutter. Many of them begin with slowing the speech to a very slow rate, even to taking an entire two seconds to say one syllable. At this slow rate, other speech goals ("targets") are often taught, such as beginning the voice in a sleepy or breathy way rather than in a crisp way. This is known as easy or gentle vocal onset. Another common target is using correct breathing, such as taking a normal, full breath before beginning to speak and using it up normally before taking another breath. A third example of a fluency shaping target is learning to move the tongue and lips as easily and lightly as possible while still preserving reasonably clear pronunciation. Ordinarily, the clinician gives the client instructions and practice in paying attention to—or monitoring—the targets as he or she talks. Then, as the various targets are mastered at a very slow rate, the speech is gradually speeded up to a more normal rate. And usually as the speed gets up to a slow normal, additional training is given to be sure that the speech sounds reasonably natural, that is, without the robotic, mechanical sound of the slower rates.

Some fluency shaping approaches include the use of various electronic devices to help clients achieve the desired targets. A few approaches utilize computer programs that record the stutterer's speech via a microphone that is connected to a computer and then essentially create "real-time acoustic biofeedback." For example, devices or programs are available where a client can look at the computer screen and see immediately—by a graph-like display—whether he has or has not produced an easy vocal onset. Another

> "I did a Hollins College kind of approach. It's a delayed voice onset, where they teach you how to start out differently; for example, instead of saying 'table,' you say 'tͪaable' to ease into it more. And it takes a lot of training." —*f, age 41*

well-known procedure called "delayed auditory feedback" involves a device that allows the stutterer to hear his own voice but in a bizarre manner. The stutterer doesn't hear what he is currently saying; rather, he hears what he said a fraction of a second earlier. For some, the result is slow speech that is free of stuttering.

Fluency shaping is sometimes called the "speak more fluently" approach. In Australia, it has been called the "prolonged speech" approach. It became popular in the 1970s and 1980s and is probably the most common type of therapy given to stutterers today. Actually, many of the techniques were used in the 1800s and early 1900s, but were dismissed early in the last century by the first specifically trained speech correctionists as distractions at best and quackery at worst. The name "fluency shaping" is most appropriately derived from an intensive therapy program called the "Precision Fluency Shaping Program" developed in the 1970s. (Annie Glenn, the wife of the astronaut and US Senator, John Glenn, was one of the program's most well-known successes.) Fluency shaping can be quite successful and can produce speech that is essentially normal to a listener. However, it generally requires a great deal of mental effort on the part of the client to maintain fluency because he must monitor his speech virtually all of the time. This is no easy task, and some stutterers who relapse (that is, go back to stuttering) after fluency shaping training do so because they find it too difficult to keep up the necessary degree of practice and the constant monitoring of speech.

> "Then I started junior high. My stuttering was still around. At this point my mother decided that the public school therapy wasn't enough. I ended up going to another speech pathologist, who did wonders for my stuttering. Initially, it was a whole bunch of tests and batteries. She decided that the treatment that was best for me required that I see her four hours a week."
>
> —*m, age 39*

Want more information?

Barry Guitar provides summaries of most of the well-known fluency shaping approaches to therapy throughout his textbook, classified according to the age and severity level of the stuttering for which they are optimally intended. Meryl Wall and Florence Myers summarize these same approaches as well but conveniently all in Chapter 8.

Guitar, B. (1998). *Stuttering: An Integrated Approach to its Nature and Treatment* (2nd Ed.). Baltimore: Williams & Wilkins.

Wall, M. J. & Myers, F. L. (1995). *Clinical Management of Childhood Stuttering* (2nd Ed.). Austin, TX: Pro-Ed.

Stuttering modification, once very popular, is undergoing a revival.

Stuttering modification—also known as the "stutter more fluently" approach—refers to a group of techniques that are designed to teach the stutterer to change the usual stuttering into an easier form of stuttering without the tension and struggle. Most of these approaches require preliminary steps of training to identify or become aware of all the core, accessory, and emotional symptoms of stuttering. Often, too, identification training is followed by desensitization techniques designed to reduce fears (see below). Once these prerequisites are achieved, three common stuttering modification techniques are taught: "cancellations," "pull-outs," and "preparatory sets." Cancellations allow the stutterer to modify his stuttering *after* it occurs by pausing, rehearsing (first out loud and then mentally) an easier "more fluent" form of stuttering on the stuttered word, then saying the word again slowly and deliberately in the more fluent way. Pull-outs basically move the process forward in time so that modification takes place *during* the stuttering. Here, as the stuttering happens, the stutterer learns to slow the repetitions, smooth out the prolongations, get something going instead of holding a block, and then slowing and deliberately *pulling out* of the old stuttering into a more fluent form. Preparatory sets essentially involve making those same adjustments mentally and perhaps physically *before* the stuttering actually comes out in the old, struggled way. One good thing about this approach is that there is always a backup procedure. If you fail with a preparatory set, you can pull-out; if you don't complete a good pull-out, you should cancel.

Stuttering modification techniques were developed during the early- and mid-1900s, but it wasn't until the '50s that the late Charles Van Riper perfected the above techniques. This approach has many names: the Van Riper approach, the traditional approach, the voluntary control approach, or the "stutter more fluently" approach. Though stuttering modification therapies were never discredited and have been employed consistently in several well-known stuttering therapy programs, many speech-language pathologists essentially replaced them during the 1960s with behavioral approaches (see below) and in the 1970s with fluency shaping

> "But what I remember is that the therapist taught me some techniques called cancellation and pull-out, and for the first time, I felt I had some control." —*m, age 56*

approaches. In the 1990s, however, stuttering modification experienced a revival, and it is currently becoming increasingly popular again, often in combination with fluency shaping. Some of the attractions for clients using stuttering modification, especially for relatively severe stutterers, are: they do not need to consider stuttering a failure, they do not need to monitor every word that is said, the speech is less likely to sound robotic than in fluency shaping, and many find that living as a controlled stutterer is psychologically more appealing than trying to pass as a normal speaker (even though that is sometimes possible). Some potential disadvantages of the approach are that it requires the ability and intelligence to anticipate and intercept stuttering, the willingness to communicate openly in spite of stuttering, and the maturity to accept regular practice of the modification techniques as a necessary life change.

Want more information?

The best source for understanding the nuances of cancellations, pull-outs, and preparatory sets is Van Riper's book itself, Chapter 12, entitled "Modification."

Van Riper, C. (1973). *The Treatment of Stuttering*. Englewood Cliffs, NJ: Prentice-Hall.

Contingent management is controversial and not widely used, but some of its principles are included in most therapies.

Contingent management approaches to treating stuttering have probably been the most controversial of all since their development and popular use in the 1960s and early 1970s. They grew out of a body of research that used "operant conditioning" procedures to investigate whether or not stuttering behaved like a habit. (Incidentally, many authorities consider these procedures to be fluency shaping, even though a careful look at the underlying rationales and methods reveals that there are marked differences in the two groups of approaches.) As I pointed out earlier, we have basically concluded that the core symptoms of stuttering cannot be explained by learning principles. But in the course of doing this research, it was found, as expected by

"I can still remember getting little treats and stickers and stars on paper for doing stuff."

—*m, age 32*

the behavioral scientists but to the dismay of many who did not subscribe to strict learning theories, that if a negative stimulus like an electric shock or obnoxious sound is delivered to the stutterer immediately after each and every stutter, the stuttering usually decreases and is sometimes eliminated. The theory began to run into trouble when it was discovered that the same reduction in stuttering happens when the stimulus is presumably "neutral," as in a simple click on a counter every time stuttering occurs, or even "positive," as in receiving a "reward" or hearing the word "good" after each stutter.

A few treatment studies tried another aversive stimulus—"time-out" from speaking—with a small number of stutterers and were successful in reducing or even eliminating stuttering in some of them. Here is how it works. As the stutterer is talking, a clinician listens and signals him to stop immediately for five to ten seconds after each and every stutter. This somehow creates an environment where the stutterer learns to speak with less and less stuttering. Other studies showed that if each period of "fluency" (or period with no stuttering) is followed by a "reward" or "reinforcer" such as a desired token or coin or the word "good," stuttering reduced as well.

A number of therapy approaches were developed which used time-out or other aversive stimuli for stuttering, rewards for fluency, or some combination of the two. Often, the stutterer would quickly become fluent, sometimes without realizing why he or she did so. That was attractive, but the results were often not as long lasting as with other approaches. Also, as I suggested above, there was a great deal of resistance to these approaches, probably because of the language originally used to describe them, namely "operant punishment." Clinicians did not want to "punish" their clients, although there was never any real evidence that stutterers felt that this kind of therapy was any worse or more difficult than other approaches. In fact, it was probably easier in many ways, because all they had to do was sit down and talk.

Due to these and other reasons, contingent management as a sole approach to stuttering therapy is not currently very popular. But the behavioral principles from these experiments in operant

"Yeah, my dad used to actually stutter. And he went to the Marine Corps in '68, '69, '70, about the time of the Vietnam War. I guess the drill instructors literally beat it out of him. I mean every time he would stutter, he'd really just get the !*#@ beat out of him." —m, age 22

conditioning are used in almost all therapies, such as counting the frequency of stuttered words or syllables as one measure of progress, and systematically and immediately rewarding the client for progress and letting him know when he makes an error. Also, contingent management is often combined with other approaches, such as fluency shaping and linguistic management (see below).

Want more information?

Jerry Siegel wrote an excellent review article thirty years ago summarizing the early operant research that had been carried out with stutterers. In it, he postulates that "highlighting" rather than "punishing" stuttering is what is responsible for the positive effects of contingent management of stuttering.

Siegel, G. M. (1970). Punishment, stuttering, and disfluency. *Journal of Speech and Hearing Research,13*, pp. 677-714.

Linguistic hierarchy management is used in most therapies.

Linguistic hierarchy management is not a well-known therapy category, but I include it here to highlight an approach that is often combined with other approaches. Essentially, it means progressing from short and easy spoken units (such as single-syllable words that are well known) to progressively longer and harder spoken units. And most often, it is combined with aspects of fluency shaping and with contingent management. (This is why some experts in fluency disorders believe that linguistic hierarchy management should be considered part of fluency shaping.) The therapy might work like this: A stutterer is first asked to read single words, one at a time. Every time he says one without stuttering, the clinician says "good" or "that's right." Every time stuttering occurs, she might say, "Try that again." Once all or nearly all the words can be read fluently, she has the stutterer read two words at a time with the same instructions. This progresses to reading aloud three to four words, to sentences, to short paragraphs, until several paragraphs can be read with little or no stuttering. Then the procedure moves to the stutterer talking about some predetermined topics (monologue), again progressing from short to longer and longer

> "She also helped me by having me read books, one word at a time, one step at a time, to slow my speech down."
>
> —*m, age 56*

utterances. After monologues are mastered, he moves straight to interactive conversations with the clinician, usually skipping the steps of one word, two words, and so on.

Linguistic hierarchy management is also used in stuttering modification and other approaches whenever a sequence from easier to more difficult speaking situations is required, both in and out of the therapy room. Its appeal is obvious. You start with the easiest material, master it, then move on to slightly more difficult material. Once that is mastered, you progress to more challenging material, and so on.

Want more information?

The section of a chapter by Bruce Ryan that describes the GILCU approach (which stands for "Gradual Increase in Length and Complexity of Utterance") is an excellent example of linguistic hierarchy management. Janis Costello Ingham also has a description of a similar program for preschool stutterers in the same book.

Ryan, B. P. (1984). Treatment of stuttering in school children. In W. H. Perkins (Ed.), *Stuttering Disorders*. pp. 95-105. New York: Thieme-Stratton.

Costello, J. A. (1984). Operant conditioning and the treatment of stuttering. In W. H. Perkins (Ed.), *Stuttering Disorders*. pp. 107-127. New York: Thieme-Stratton.

Desensitization and counseling, once quite popular, are also undergoing a revival.

As we have noted, stuttering is unpleasant and is associated with lots of troubling thoughts and feelings. Desensitization and counseling are designed to help the stutterer overcome or manage emotions and thoughts associated with stuttering. Some experts might separate dealing with thoughts as "cognitive" approaches, but the overlap with dealing with emotions is so great that I chose to combine them here.

Desensitization is a term that Van Riper borrowed (and changed slightly) to describe the process of learning to reduce or manage the negative emotions associated with stuttering. Some

"The more experience you have in times that you previously stuttered, like in front of the class, you would begin to become relaxed and realize that you are OK, and that you'll be all right. You gain confidence after two or three speeches or presentations, and you begin to forget about it."

—*m, age 22*

refer to this approach as nonavoidance. Among other things, it includes a wide variety of techniques that help a person confront and overcome his fears of stuttering. One common technique is to learn to stutter on purpose (fake stuttering) to strangers in real or realistic contrived speaking situations. The suggestion to go out and stutter on purpose usually creates a great deal of anxiety and resistance in the stutterer. But when—with the clinician's support and guidance—he has summoned up the courage to talk to a few dozen strangers using even one easy faked stutter per situation along with his usual real stutters, a great burden of fear as frequently experienced is lifted from his shoulders. Suddenly, it is as if the stutterer's worst fear becomes manageable. How, indeed, can one avoid and hide stuttering while going out and advertising it? Another technique is learning to speak assertively while maintaining normal eye contact with a person while stuttering. Nothing communicates confidence and self-acceptance to a listener more effectively than looking him squarely in the eye while conversing with him. Once achieved, this also gives the speaker a healthy sense of power. The stutterer discovers it is possible to do all of these even while stuttering. Numerous other techniques, including role playing, experiencing the liberating power of humor, and sharing feelings with others, can be effective desensitization techniques as well.

Unloading one's fears and painful experiences in a safe environment is highly therapeutic as well. The good clinician creates such an environment and allows the stutterer to experience a cleansing and catharsis. And, to the extent that her training allows, she provides counseling and guidance to the stutterer as he comes to grip with a long history of avoidance, social embarrassment, fear, and compromised self esteem.

The benefits of being able to manage the negative feelings and thoughts are obvious. But are they necessary? Clinicians whose approaches consist primarily of changing or normalizing the

> "What I do remember is that one of my father's big things was, he made me participate in the plays all of the time. So I was constantly in school plays where I had to read in front of people. And then I had to be a narrator for the plays, and then I had to read in church. That was his big thing, because he thought it was a confidence thing. I think in some ways he might have been right because I had to do all those things constantly, and by the time I had gotten to the fourth grade, there was nothing there. Even when I got nervous, I really wouldn't even stutter." —m, age 32

stuttering might argue that if I can make you fluent, the feelings will take care of themselves. Most stutterers would agree. To the extent that learning and maintaining fluent speech over several years is possible, there probably is no need to do lots of desensitization. However, the attempts of the behavioral therapists of the '60s and fluency shaping therapists of the '70s, '80s, and '90s to manage the stuttering only, resulted in the persistence of emotional baggage and probably contributed as much to relapses as lack of skill development did. For this reason, since the mid-'90s, a revival of desensitization in therapy has taken place. Whatever approach might be used to change the speech pattern, many clinicians are now dealing specifically with fears, shame, and guilt, even in young children who stutter.

Working with preschool-aged stutterers is, of course, different from working with older children and adults. In the case of desensitization, the child's parents mediate much of the effort. Parents are taught to reduce speech-related pressures and to help their child express his or her feelings about stuttering directly and through play. Clinicians often provide settings to allow them to come to grips with their own feelings of frustration, pain, and guilt regarding their child's stuttering. Finally, they are often taught to be partners in speech therapy, helping to carry out other techniques in the home, such as modeling slow and easy speech to the child.

Want more information?

Again one of the best sources for understanding desensitization is Van Riper's book, Chapter 11, entitled "Desensitization."

Van Riper, C. (1973). *The Treatment of Stuttering*. Englewood Cliffs, NJ: Prentice-Hall.

Also, two other sources are worth mentioning for counseling. Walt Manning and David Shapiro both provide compelling and clear descriptions of several individual counseling techniques in their books. Shapiro adds an interesting review of family systems and their relationship to stuttering.

Manning, W. H. (2001). *Clinical Decision Making in Fluency Disorders* (2nd Ed.). San Diego, CA: Singular.

Shapiro, D. A. (1999). *Stuttering Intervention: A Collaborative Journey to Fluency Freedom*. Austin, TX: Pro-Ed.

Staying fluent is as important as getting fluent.

Let us now address a few issues that pertain to all approaches to therapy. I tell my students and clients that there are two problems in stuttering therapy: getting fluent ("establishment") and staying fluent ("transfer and maintenance"). I realize that this distinction might seem as trite as the advice a manager might give to his boxer, "There are only two things to watch out for, his right and his left!" But, getting fluent is a different problem than staying fluent, though it is certainly a prerequisite.

Most therapies now have both a transfer and maintenance component. Transfer means becoming and staying fluent with other people and in other settings during the standard period of therapy visits. The most astute clinicians do not assume that if a person is fluent in a session he or she will be equally fluent in other settings. Therefore, once the skills are learned in a one-on-one situation, therapy involves getting out of the safety of the therapy room and into the real world: talking to friends and co-workers, making telephone calls, interacting with store-keepers and people on the street and so on.

Maintenance involves staying fluent with other people in other settings over several years. In order to achieve this, it is important for the stutterer to continue practicing, monitoring, lessening fears, etc. for a long time after formal therapy is finished. Some of the activities (depending on the approach to therapy) that might be suggested include such things as: a daily regimen of a few minutes of practice, voluntary stuttering once a week, attending a self-help group for five years (see below), becoming one's own therapist, or recognizing and dealing with a relapse.

> "We did things like she would make me call Pizza Hut and order. Or she would call me on the telephone just any time of the day or the week-end—she was wonderful! —and make me talk to her. Or she would make me call. I remember her making me make so many phone calls a day and making a recording of it, and that kind of thing. So that helped me more because I think mine was really triggered by anxieties, I really do."
>
> —f, age 27

Want more information?

David Shapiro provides a number of excellent suggestions for procedures that can be used to foster transfer and maintenance at various age levels.

Shapiro, D. A. (1999). *Stuttering Intervention: A Collaborative Journey to Fluency Freedom*. Austin, TX: Pro-Ed.

Most therapy involves regular visits over months or years; some involves intensive work over a few weeks.

Another general issue concerns the time frame of therapy. Most therapy that is carried out in public school, hospital, or clinic settings uses the familiar "come in once or twice a week model." This kind of "extended" model certainly has its advantages, but truthfully the biggest reason it is used seems to be that it is most familiar; it is, after all, how clinicians were trained. But the "intensive" model, though much less widespread, has been used for many years as well. In the limited programs that use an intensive model, a group of clients all begin and go through therapy together all day, every day for a period of two to three weeks. These programs are more likely to specialize in stuttering instead of providing therapy for stuttering along with the gamut of other speech and language disorders.

Perhaps the biggest advantage of the extended model is that it fits more easily into the stutterer's work, school, or family routine. Because sessions are spread out over time, costs may be more manageable for clients or families who are paying themselves, or they may be more in line with a medical insurance plan's policies and restrictions. The main disadvantage of extended therapy is that progress is often slow. Sometimes, the client loses interest before he sees the change he desires. By contrast, the main advantage of the intensive model is that stutterers generally are highly successful in a short time. Positive energy and optimism from the group typically enhance success and motivation. Also, as I hinted above, it is more likely that stuttering specialists will be involved with this kind of therapy. The main disadvantage of the intensive model is that many stutterers find it hard to maintain their gains over a long period of time without the ongoing support of the clinician or the other stutterers in the group. Thus, relapse and the shocking disappointment that goes

"The sessions were long and I had homework to do for her on top of my school assignments. It was rough, but eventually it was slowly but surely helping. She taught me to monitor everything I said. At first it was hard to do, but I got used to it after only six months. It was weird, but it just clicked. During the sessions we didn't do 'fun' stuff like we did in school sessions. I did a lot of listening to myself. She'd tape me and do all sorts of crazy things with the tape. We'd always talk for a half hour about things like what was going on in school. I worked with her all through sixth grade, seventh, eighth and periodically through ninth. *(continued next page)*

along with it are not uncommon. Though intensive therapy may seem very expensive, if you count all the hours of help received, it may actually cost much less than an equivalent amount of therapy in the extended model.

One model that has been explored, but not utilized as much as it could be, is a combination of the intensive and extended models. I once developed and briefly ran such a model wherein elementary school-aged stutterers were helped to become very fluent in a two-week summer intensive program at a private clinic specializing in stuttering and then assisted by their school clinicians over the next year or two for half-hour sessions twice a week, then once a week, to help them stay fluent. Unfortunately, I was unable to continue the program. Similar models, if they could be coordinated and maintained, would hold particular promise for stutterers who had not responded well to the usual available models.

...the sessions got shorter and shorter, and then finally she told me that I'd graduated from speech therapy after ten years!! I mean, I can't get rid of my stutter, but I speak pretty fluently for someone who stuttered as bad as I did. I haven't actually had any speech therapy since I was fourteen and all, but I know everything there is to know about stuttering. I lived it."

—m, age 39

Want more information?

I co-authored a chapter a number of years ago that summarized this issue of models of therapy and a number of other issues related to the effectiveness of stuttering therapy.

St. Louis, K. O. & Westbrook, J. B. (1987). The effectiveness of treatment for stuttering. In L. Rustin, H. Purser, & D. Rowley (Eds.), *Progress in the Treatment of Fluency Disorders*. pp. 235-257. London: Taylor & Francis.

Self-help or support groups are becoming more and more available.

Another very important issue concerns the self-help or support group movement for stuttering, which is becoming an increasingly available and important component of managing stuttering. A support group movement for stuttering was essentially nonexistent until the 1970s. Gains were slow through the 1980s but currently, the self-help movement is healthy and growing rapidly. The largest group in the US is the National Stuttering Association (formerly, the National Stuttering Project), which provides assistance and guidance to individual self-help and support group chapters all over the country. Of course, aspects of self-management and therapy come into play in these groups. Regular meetings of stutterers and other interested persons provide ongoing support for individuals, regardless of their needs. Some go to self-help groups to practice and maintain their gains from speech therapy; some attend because they have no interest in formal speech therapy yet seek the therapeutic support of others; some enjoy a chance to socialize in a non-threatening and understanding environment; still others become regular members to help and guide others. In addition to meeting the needs of its members (such as hosting an annual national convention), the National Stuttering Association has started to provide continuing education for speech-language pathologists who seek to know more about treating stuttering.

Want more information?

Lee Reeves, who has been a leader in the National Stuttering Association, wrote an excellent article on how self-help or support groups can be useful in managing stuttering.

Reeves, L. (1998). *The role of self-help/support groups in determining the outcomes of stuttering therapy.* Paper presented at the International Stuttering Awareness Day On-Line Conference. http://www.mankato.msus.edu/dept/comdis/isad/papers/reeves.html.

A few formally recognized Specialists in Fluency Disorders are now available.

Finally, let me briefly discuss an issue that I mentioned earlier in this chapter, namely specialization in stuttering therapy. In the past decade, training for students studying speech-language pathology in universities in the US has diminished in the area of stuttering. There are a number of reasons for this; let me highlight two. First,

"They also had bi-monthly local chapter meetings of the National Stuttering Association. The group was more structured. It was just people getting together and talking and just practicing talking. That's all there is to it. And I was thinking, 'Hmm, this is a little private. I don't know if I want to listen to this.' But I did, and he was asking her about how she felt about herself because she stuttered. She said that she felt that people wouldn't think that she was as much as she was. They would, you know, kind of look down on her. Think she was incompetent, incapable, and all this. And when I saw that, I was like, 'You know, that's exactly how I felt.'"

—m, age 22

the American Speech-Language-Hearing Association (ASHA) has established requirements for awarding Certification of Clinical Competence in Speech-Language Pathology (CCC/SLP). This is a nationally recognized professional designation, and indicates, for example (among other things), that an individual has completed master's level studies at an "ASHA approved" university training program. In 1992, ASHA eliminated hands-on practice treating stuttering from the CCC/SLP requirements. Behind this change was pressure from directors of university training programs who found it difficult to assure the requisite twenty-five hours of hands-on practicum in fluency disorders for every student. Currently, many new speech-language pathologists graduating with master's degrees have had no hands-on experience with stuttering.

> "I went to a speech therapist in high school, and I didn't really like what she was doing. She would make me talk and clap my hands at the same time. Trying to get into a rhythm so I didn't stutter, and I just didn't like what she was doing. I felt like a seal in Sea World waiting for her to feed me fish after I clapped my hands. So I didn't like doing that, and I just stopped going on my own." —*m, age 33*

As a result, there has been an ongoing problem of clinicians feeling insecure about—and therefore reluctant toward—treating stuttering. The reasons behind this are complex, but I have speculated that one big reason relates to a responsibility issue. Compared to other speech or language disorders, clinicians recognize that stutterers could become essentially normal if the right therapy is used successfully. That places a lot of pressure on the clinician, and many don't want to shoulder that responsibility, especially after one or two of their clients have relapsed. Of course, providing *less* training to students is no way to help alleviate their insecurity and reluctance!

The second reason that training in stuttering has diminished is that the field of speech-language pathology has grown rapidly in other areas. This has required additional training in such areas as clinical applications of technology for nonspeaking individuals and collaboration with other medical professionals to evaluate and assist with feeding and swallowing problems of specialized patients. Consequently, what were once required courses in fluency disorders are now offered as one of many optional speech-language pathology electives for students, and in some cases, such courses have been dropped altogether.

Interestingly, these changes in professional training have happened as the self-help and support movement in stuttering has experienced unprecedented growth. Knowledge and expectations among stutterers is increasing while knowledge and expertise in stuttering treatment among most speech-language pathologists is decreasing. To deal with this growing problem, ASHA's Special Interest Division 4 on Fluency and Fluency Disorders established a new Specialty Board on Fluency Disorders in 1999 whose mission is to develop and administer a "Specialty Recognition in Fluency Disorders" program. I was fortunate to serve on the first Board, which evaluated and brought about 300 specialists into the program. As this program grows, it is likely that these "Board Recognized Specialists" will be sought to treat stuttering and to provide training to other generalist speech-language pathologists who find themselves needing to treat stuttering clients. Our hope is that, over time, stuttering treatment will be dramatically improved as a result of this innovative program.

> "And also what's, I guess, what's good about this day and age, is you can get specialists who will help you on this, but back then they may have had them, but heck my family could not afford it." —*m, age 60*

How can stutterers be more successful?

Let me end my discussion of management of stuttering with six suggestions that could enhance the likelihood of success in managing stuttering.

> "If I have any friends, I'll just tell them straight— straight to them that they should take their kid to the therapist right away and get it cleared up at a young age. Then in the future everything should be OK." —*m, age 23*

Start early if you can.

Refer or take a youngster who is stuttering to a speech-language pathologist as soon as possible. The evidence is clear. The younger the child, the better the chances for a complete "cure" for stuttering with speech therapy. Of course, we know that the large majority of preschoolers would recover spontaneously with no therapy, but even those who would not still seem to respond best to early therapy. Why? The answer is not entirely clear, but we suspect that the habits that grow up around stuttering are not strong in beginning stutterers and that they have not yet acquired the devastating self-esteem problems that stutterers with years of experience have. If you are an adult who stutters and did not have the benefit of early therapy, this suggestion no doubt has come too late to cure your stuttering. Still, there are all kinds of reasons to be hopeful. If that is your case, read on!

Get good advice and help.

If possible, arrange to talk to a Board Recognized Specialist in Fluency Disorders about your stuttering. If that is impossible, consult with a speech-language pathologist who has expressed an interest in treating stuttering and who has taken graduate-level coursework in the subject. If that cannot be done, try contacting the Stuttering Foundation of America and the National Stuttering Association for resources they might recommend. Finally, in the absence of any luck there, try contacting your closest university training program in speech-language pathology for recommendations. *Appendix C: How and where you can get help for your stuttering* provides resources that can help you locate specialists, self-help groups, and materials.

Don't try too hard *not to stutter.*

This advice might not be relevant if you stutter and have never had any speech therapy. But, if you are in speech therapy or have had it in the past, be aware that using the techniques to try very hard never to stutter is often a blueprint for eventual disappointment. Even if you learned the techniques correctly, if your main motivation is never to stutter, chances are that you will not experience their benefits or will sooner or later relapse. Try this advice instead. *Try to talk in a new way and let the stuttering take care of itself.* Stuttering (or stuttering in the old way) may not be what you are striving for, but these "failures" can be turned into successes if you calmly analyze what went wrong and think about what you can do in terms of speaking skills to fix it.

Have courage.

Never underestimate the power of facing up to a difficult situation. If you can muster the courage to go to a self-help group for the first time, or to go to therapy, or to tell someone you stutter, or to stutter on purpose, you have already succeeded in a major way. Managing confirmed stuttering is not for the faint of heart and does require courage. Don't worry if you feel anxious or scared, you can learn to act in spite of those feelings, and, over time, those actions will reduce the fear.

Be determined.

As the stories in this book make clear, setbacks and relapses occur in most cases of successful management of stuttering. It is important to realize that your eventual success will inevitably involve some failures along the way. Also, remember that, except for young children who often succeed without knowing why, most older stutterers have to make a few serious lifestyle changes in order to consistently manage their stuttering. If you have learned that you must make such changes, it is your determination to stay focused that will lead you to success. One of the best ways to do this is to follow your clinician's advice if you are in therapy. If you are not enrolled in therapy, attending and participating actively in a support group is the sort of discipline that can keep you on track for the rest of your life.

Try to be optimistic and to have a healthy sense of humor.

Along with courage and determination, optimism is an important ingredient in achieving success over stuttering. If you believe you can, your chances are far greater than if you believe you cannot. And if you can proceed with a smile on your face, so much the better. Of course, stuttering is basically not funny, but the stutterers I've met who

"In some ways stuttering has made me who I am. It gave me a grit and determination I might not otherwise have." —m, age 45

"It rarely happens when I am in the classroom teaching. I guess I have all the confidence in the world when I am up there performing for my students. So if anything, if I do pause or have some stutter, I use humor to break it up a little bit and make some comment about my false teeth, or being tongue-tied by the beauty of the girl in the third seat, or some other way to cover it up." —m, age 59

can laugh at themselves feel least like victims. A sense of humor and optimism are contagious; the more you have, the more other people will help you out, give you a break, and cheer you on.

Keep stuttering in its proper perspective.

How much should stuttering determine our outlook and our choices? No one can tell you what role stuttering should play in you life. I suffered from stuttering a great deal as a youth, but it led me to my life's work. That's good. On the other hand, I still avoid making calls sometimes if I can and miss more life experiences than I need to. In an ideal world, stuttering would have little impact on our life's choices. After all, we *can* talk (stutteringly sometimes), we do have things worth listening to, we have myriad other skills, and we want for our loved ones and ourselves the same kinds of things other people do.

If you don't know the answer to the question, "How much does stuttering determine your outlook and choices?" I suggest you "take stock" of your stuttering as presented in *Appendices C, G,* and *H.* I predict that you will see some interesting ways and changes in the role that stuttering has played in your life. Just as I have, you may discover some unrecognized progress, as well as some areas where you have more work to do.

"**Stuttering is not even in my top ten problems now.**" —*m, age 56*

Appendices

Ahlbach, J. & Benson, V. (1994). *To Say What is Ours.* Anaheim Hills, CA: National Stuttering Project.

American Speech-Language-Hearing Association. (1994, March). Code of ethics. *Asha, 36* (Suppl. 13), pp. 1-2.

American Speech-Language-Hearing Association, Clinical Certification Board. (1994). Chapter III: Standards and implementations for the certificates of clinical competence. In Clinical Certification Board, *Membership and Certification Handbook: Speech-Language Pathology– 1995*, pp. 7-17.

American Speech-Language-Hearing Association, Special Interest Division 4: Fluency and Fluency Disorders. (1995, March). Guidelines for practice in stuttering treatment. *Asha, 37* (Suppl. 14), pp. 26-35.

American Speech-Language-Hearing Association, Special Interest Division 4: Fluency and Fluency Disorders. (1999, March). Terminology pertaining to fluency and fluency disorders: Guidelines. *Asha, 41* (Suppl. 19), pp. 29-36.

Baumeister, R. F. & Newman, L. S. (1994). How stories make sense of personal experiences: Motives that shape autobiographical narratives. *Personality and Social Psychology Bulletin, 20*, pp. 676-690.

Baumgartner, J. M. (1999). Acquired psychogenic stuttering. In R. F. Curlee (Ed.), *Stuttering and Related Disorders of Fluency* (2nd Ed.), pp. 269-288. New York: Thieme.

Bernstein Ratner, N. E. (1997). Leaving Las Vegas: Clinical odds and individual outcomes. *American Journal of Speech-Lanuage Pathology, 6*, pp. 29-33.

Blood, G. (2000). *The stigma of stuttering: Centuries of negative perceptions and stereotypes.* Paper presented at the Annual Convention of the American Speech-Language-Hearing Association. Washington, DC.

Bloodstein, O. (1995). *A Handbook on Stuttering* (5th Ed.). San Diego, CA: Singular.

Bloom, C. & Cooperman, D. K. (1999). *Synergistic Stuttering Therapy: A Holistic Approach.* Boston: Butterworth-Heinemann.

Chmela, K. A. & Reardon, N. A. (1997). *The School-age Child Who Stutters: Working Effectively with Attitudes and Emotions.* Video and booklet. Memphis, TN: Stuttering Foundation of America.

Conture, E. G. (2001). *Stuttering: Its Nature, Diagnosis, and Treatment* (3rd Ed.). Boston: Allyn & Bacon.

Costello, J. A. (1984). Operant conditioning and the treatment of stuttering. In W. H. Perkins (Ed.), *Stuttering Disorders*, pp. 107-127. New York: Thieme-Stratton.

Cox, M. D. (1986). The psychologically maladjusted stutterer. In K. O. St. Louis (Ed.), *The Atypical Stutterer*, pp. 65-91. New York: Academic Press.

Curlee, R. F. (Ed.). (1999). *Stuttering and Related Disorders of Fluency* (2nd Ed.). New York: Thieme.

Curlee, R. F. & Siegel, G. M. (Eds.). (1997). *Nature and Treatment of Stuttering: New Directions* (2nd Ed.). Needham Heights, MA: Allyn & Bacon.

Curlee, R. F. & Yairi, E. (1997). Early intervention with early childhood stuttering: A critical examination of the data. *American Journal of Speech-Language Pathology*, 6, pp. 8-18.

Daly, D. A. (1996). *The Source for Stuttering and Cluttering*. East Moline, IL: LinguiSystems.

De Nil, L. F. (1999). Stuttering: A neurophysiological perspective. In N. Bernstein Ratner & E. C. Healey (Eds.), *Stuttering Research and Practice: Bridging the Gap*, pp. 85-102. Mahwah, NJ: Erlbaum.

Eisenson, J. (1958). A perseverative theory of stuttering. In J. Eisenson (Ed.), *Stuttering: A Symposium*, pp. 225-271. New York: Harper & Row.

Frankl, V. E. (1959). *Man's Search for Meaning: An Introduction to Logotherapy*. New York: Washington Square Press.

Freund, H. (1966). *Psychopathology and the Problems of Stuttering*. Springfield, IL: Thomas.

Goebel, M., Hillis, J., & Meyer, R. (1987). *The relationship between speech fluency and certain patterns of speech flow.* Paper presented at the annual convention of the American Speech-Language-Hearing Association, Washington, DC.

Guitar, B. (1998). *Stuttering: An Integrated Approach to its Nature and Treatment* (2nd Ed.). Baltimore: Williams & Wilkins.

Ham, R. E. (1999). *Clinical Management of Stuttering in Older Children and Adults*. Gaithersburg, MD: Aspen.

Haroldson, S. K., Martin, R. R., & Starr, C. D. (1968). Time-out as a punishment for stuttering. *Journal of Speech and Hearing Research, 11*, pp. 560-566.

Helm-Estabrooks, N. (1999). Stuttering associated with acquired neurological disorders. In R. F. Curlee (Ed.), *Stuttering and Related Disorders of Fluency* (2nd Ed.), pp. 255-268. New York: Thieme.

Hoagland, E. (2001). The football game in my head. In *U.S. News & World Report* (April 2, 2001), pp. 50-51.

Ingham, R. J. (1984). *Stuttering and Behavior Therapy: Current Status and Experimental Foundations*. San Diego, CA: College-Hill Press.

Ingham, R. J. (1998). On learning from speech-motor control research on stuttering. In A. K. Cordes & R. J. Ingham (Eds.), *Treatment Efficacy for Stuttering: A Search for Empirical Bases*, pp. 67-101. San Diego, CA: Singular.

Jezer, M. (1997). *Stuttering: A Life Bound up in Words*. New York: BasicBooks.

Johnson, W. & Associates. (1959). *The Onset of Stuttering: Research Findings and Implications*. Minneapolis: The University of Minnesota Press.

Kloth, S., Janssen, P., Kraaimaat, F., & Brutten, G. J. (1998). Child and mother variables in the development of stuttering among high-risk children: A longitudinal study. *Journal of Fluency Disorders, 23,* pp. 217-230.

Kolk, H. & Postma, A. (1997). Stuttering as a covert repair phenomenon. In R. F. Curlee & G. M. Siegel (Eds.), *Nature and Treatment of Stuttering: New Directions* (2nd Ed.), pp. 182-203. New York: Allyn & Bacon.

Langevin, M. (1997). Peer teasing project. In E. Healey & H. F. M. Peters (Eds.), *Proceedings of the Second World Congress on Fluency Disorders,* pp. 169-171. The Netherlands: Nijmegen University Press.

Langevin, M. (2000). *Teasing and Bullying: Unacceptable Behaviour.* Edmonton, Alberta: The Institute for Stuttering Treatment and Research.

Mandler, J. M. (1984). *Stories, Scripts, and Scenes: Aspects of Schema Theory.* Hillsdale, NJ: Lawrence Erlbaum Associates.

Manning, W. H. (2001). *Clinical Decision Making in Fluency Disorders* (2nd Ed.). San Diego, CA: Singular.

Martin, R. R., Kuhl, P., & Haroldson, S. (1972). An experimental treatment with two preschool stuttering children. *Journal of Speech Hearing Research, 15,* pp. 743-752.

Monk, G., Winslade, J., Crocket, K., & Epston, D. (Eds.). (1997). *Narrative Therapy in Practice: The Archaeology of Hope.* San Francisco: Jossey-Bass Publishers.

Murphy, B. (1999). A preliminary look at shame, guilt, and stuttering. In N. Bernstein Ratner & E. C. Healey (Eds.), *Stuttering Research and Practice: Bridging the Gap,* pp. 131-143. Mahwah, NJ: Erlbaum.

Murray, F. P. (1991). *A Stutterer's Story.* Memphis, TN: Stuttering Foundation of America.

Myers, F. L., & St. Louis, K. O. (Eds.). (1992). *Cluttering: A Clinical Perspective.* Leicester: FAR Communications. Reissued 1996: San Diego, CA: Singular.

Nietzsche, F. (1968). *Twilight of the Idols.* R. J. Hollingdale, Translator. Harmondsworth, Middlesex, England: Penguin Books. (Original work published 1889.)

Onslow, M. (1996). *Behavioral Management of Stuttering.* San Diego, CA: Singular.

Parry, A., & Doan, R. E. (1994). *Story Re-visions: Narrative Therapy in the Postmodern World.* New York: The Guilford Press.

Progoff, I. (1975). *At a Journal Workshop: The Basic Text and Guide for Using the Intensive Journal® Process.* New York: Dialogue House Library.

Quesal, R. W. (1998). Knowledge, understanding, and acceptance. In E. C. Healey & H. F. M. Peters (Eds.), *Proceedings of the Second World Congress on Fluency Disorders,* pp. 384-387. The Netherlands: Nijmegen University Press.

Rainer, T. (1997). *Your Life as Story: Discovering the "New Autobiography" and Writing Memoir as Literature.* New York: Tarcher/Putnam.

Reeves, L. (1998). *The role of self-help/support groups in determining the outcomes of stuttering therapy.* Paper presented at the International Stuttering Awareness Day On-Line Conference. http://www.mankato.msus.edu/dept/comdis/isad/papers/reeves.html.

Ryan, B. P. (1974). *Programmed Therapy for Stuttering in Children and Adults.* Springfield, IL: Thomas.

Ryan, B. P. (1984). Treatment of stuttering in school children. In W. H. Perkins (Ed.), *Stuttering Disorders,* pp. 95-105. New York: Thieme-Stratton.

Shapiro, D. A. (1999). *Stuttering Intervention: A Collaborative Journey to Fluency Freedom.* Austin, TX: Pro-Ed.

Sheehan, J. G. (1970). Role therapy. In J. G. Sheehan (Ed.), *Stuttering Research and Therapy,* pp. 261-310. New York: Harper & Row.

Siegel, G. M. (1970). Punishment, stuttering, and disfluency. *Journal of Speech and Hearing Research, 13,* pp. 677-714.

Smith, A. & Kelly, E. (1997). Stuttering: A dynamic, multifactorial model. In R. F. Curlee & G. M. Siegel (Eds.), *Nature and Treatment of Stuttering: New Directions* (2nd Ed.), pp. 204-217. Needham Heights, MA: Allyn & Bacon.

Sobel, R. K. (2001). Anatomy of a stutterer. In *U.S. News & World Report* (April 2, 2001), pp. 44-51.

Specialty Board on Fluency Disorders. (2001). *Specialty Board on Fluency Disorders Manual.* Memphis, TN.

Starkweather, C. W. & Givens-Ackerman, J. (1997). *Stuttering.* Austin, TX: Pro-Ed.

St. Louis, K. O. (1979). Linguistic and motor aspects of stuttering. In N. J. Lass (Ed.), *Speech and Language: Advances in Basic Research and Practice,* Vol. 1, pp. 89-210. New York: Academic Press.

St. Louis, K. O. (1997). What is stuttering: Some more current additions. In S. B. Hood (Ed.), *Stuttering Words,* p. 12. Memphis, TN: Stuttering Foundation of America.

St. Louis, K. O. (1998). *Cluttering: Some Guidelines.* Memphis, TN: Stuttering Foundation of America.

St. Louis, K. O. (1998). Your life is too important to spend it worrying about stuttering. In S. B. Hood (Ed.), *Advice for Those Who Stutter* (No. 9, 2nd Ed.), pp. 141-145. Memphis, TN: Stuttering Foundation of America.

St. Louis, K. O. (1999). Person-first labeling and stuttering. *Journal of Fluency Disorders, 24,* pp. 1-24.

St. Louis, K. O. & Durrenberger, C. H. (1993). What communication disorders do experienced clinicians prefer to manage? *Asha, 35* (December), pp. 23-31, 35.

St. Louis, K. O. & Myers, F. L. (1997). Management of cluttering and related fluency disorders. In R. F. Curlee and G. M. Siegel (Eds.), *Nature and Treatment of Stuttering: New Directions* (2nd Ed.), pp. 313-332. New York: Allyn & Bacon.

St. Louis, K. O., Ruscello, D. M., & Lundeen, C. (1992). Coexistence of communication disorders in schoolchildren. *Asha Monograph*, No. 27.

St. Louis, K. O. & Westbrook, J. B. (1987). The effectiveness of treatment for stuttering. In L. Rustin, H. Purser, & D. Rowley (Eds.), *Progress in the Treatment of Fluency Disorders*, pp. 235-257. London: Taylor & Francis.

St. Louis, K. O., Yaruss, J. S., Lubker, B. B., Pill, J., & Diggs, C. C. (2001). An international public opinion survey of stuttering: Pilot results. In H-G. Bosshardt, J. S. Yaruss, & H. F. M. Peters (Eds.), Fluency disorders: Theory, research, treatment and self-help. *Proceedings of the Third World Congress on Fluency Disorders in Nyborg, Denmark*, pp. 581-587. International Fluency Association.

St. Louis, M. J. (1996). *Put It In Writing: Guide for Populore Narratives*. Morgantown, WV: Populore.

Travis, L. E. (1957). The unspeakable feeling of people, with special reference to stuttering. In L. E. Travis (Ed.), *Handbook of Speech Pathology*, pp. 916-946, New York: Appelton-Century-Crofts.

Van Riper, C. (1973). *The Treatment of Stuttering*. Englewood Cliffs, NJ: Prentice-Hall.

Van Riper, C. (1982). *The Nature of Stuttering* (2nd Ed.). Englewood Cliffs, NJ: Prentice-Hall.

Wall, M. J. & Myers, F. L. (1995). *Clinical Management of Childhood Stuttering* (2nd Ed.). Austin, TX: Pro-Ed.

Walton, P. & Wallace, M. (1998). *Fun with Fluency: Direct Therapy with the Young Child*. Bisbee, AZ: Imaginart International.

Webster, R. L. (1980). Evolution of a target-based behavioral therapy for stuttering. *Journal of Fluency Disorders, 5*, pp. 303-320.

White, M. (1989). The externalizing of the problem and reauthoring of lives and relationships. In M. White, *Selected Papers*, p. 6. Adelaide, Australia: Dulwich Centre Publications.

White, M. & Epston, D. (1990). *Narrative Means to Therapeutic Ends*. New York: Norton.

Yaruss, J. S. (1998). Describing the consequences of disorders: Stuttering and the international classification of impairments, disabilities, and handicaps. *Journal of Speech, Language, and Hearing Research, 42*, pp. 249-257.

Zebrowski, P. M. (1997). Assisting young children who stutter and their families: Defining the role of the speech-language pathologist. *American Journal of Speech-Language Pathology, 6*, pp. 19-28.

For adults who stutter

If you want to spend only 10 minutes...

Did you know...Fact sheet about stuttering. Memphis, TN: Stuttering Foundation of America. (Brochure: #47, www.stutteringhelp.org, 1-800-992-9392)

How to react when speaking with someone who stutters. Memphis, TN: Stuttering Foundation of America. (Brochure: #46, www.stutteringhelp.org, 1-800-992-9392, Spanish version: #63)

If you want to spend 30 minutes...

Do you stutter: Straight talk for teens. Memphis, TN: Stuttering Foundation of America. (Videotape: 30 minutes, www.stutteringhelp.org, 1-800-992-9392)

If you want to spend 2 hours...

St. Louis, K. O. (Ed.). (2001). *Living with Stuttering: Stories, Basics, Resources, and Hope.* Morgantown, WV: Populore Publishing Company. (1-866-667-8679)

If you want to spend 1 day, read/watch the above materials plus...

If you stutter: Advice for adults. Memphis, TN: Stuttering Foundation of America. (Videotape: 60 minutes, www.stutteringhelp.org, 1-800-992-9392)

If you think your child is stuttering.... Memphis, TN: Stuttering Foundation of America. (Brochure: #41, www.stutteringhelp.org, 1-800-992-9392, Spanish version: #48)

Parry, W. D. (1988). *Being your own best advocate* (from *Letting Go,* September 1998). (Brochure: www.nsastutter.org, 1-800-364-1677)

Browse Judy Kuster's "The Stuttering Homepage" http://www.stutteringhomepage.com

If you want to spend 5 days, read/watch the above materials plus...

Bondarenko, V. *Voices to remember* (Videotape: 60 minutes. US—Suncoast Media, 2938 West Bay Dr., Suite B, Belleair Bluffs, FL 34640; Canada—Magic Lantern Communications, 775 Pacific Road, Oakville, ONT L6L 6M4)

Jezer, M. *(1997). Stuttering: A Life Bound up in Words*. New York: Basic Books

Hood, S. B. (Ed.). (2000). *Advice to those who stutter* (2nd Ed.). Memphis, TN: Stuttering Foundation of America. (Book: #9, www.stutteringhelp.org; 1-800-992-9392)

Browse through and read several articles from the 1st (1998), 2nd (1999), and 3rd (2000) International Stuttering Awareness Day (ISAD) On-Line Conferences. These were papers submitted electronically to "conferences" that began on October 1st each year and ended about three weeks later. During each conference, individuals anywhere who had access to the World Wide Web were able to post questions or comments that could be answered or responded to by authors or other interested persons. Consider, especially, the following papers:

from 1998 (http://www.mankato.msus.edu/dept/comdis/isad/isadcon.html):

Paths toward recovery, featuring a panel of Kristin Chmela (Illinois, US), Geoff Johnston (South Australia), Walt Manning (Tennessee, US) and Bob Quesal (Illinois, US)

Adolescents who stutter: the urgent need for support groups (A parent's perspective) by Lee Caggiano (New York, US)

Consumer self-help and professional associations by Charlie Diggs (Maryland, US)

Stuttering Foundation of America — Looking back and looking forward by Jane Fraser (Tennessee, US)

Enhancements to integrated approaches for treating stuttering by E. Charles Healey (Nebraska, US), Janet Norris (Louisiana, US), Lisa Scott Trautman (Kansas, US), and Michael Susca (Nebraska, US)

Speaking is my challenge — And I'm facing up to it by Marty Jezer (Vermont, US)

What is "successful" stuttering therapy? by Robert Quesal (Illinois, US)

The role of self-help/support groups in determining the outcomes of stuttering therapy by Lee Reeves (Texas, US)

Relapse: A misnomer? by C. Woodruff Starkweather (Pennsylvania, US)

A model for change from a consumer's perspective by Michael Sugarman (California, US)

from 1999 (http://www.mankato.msus.edu/dept/comdis/isad2/isadcon2.html):

Public speaking for stutterers by Russ Hicks (Texas, US)

Stuttering: The real world by Michael Hughes (Canada)

Creating your own map for change by Walter Manning (Tennessee, US)

Stuttering and employment discrimination by William Parry (US)

Change by David Preece (United Kingdom)

"One size fits all (or: When the only tool you have is a hammer...)" by Bob Quesal (Illinois, US)

Voluntary stuttering—when, how, and for what purpose by Andreas Starke (Germany)

The stutterer's experience by C. Woodruff Starkweather (Pennsylvania, US)

Overview and brief history of the National Stuttering Association by Michael Sugarman (California, US)

from 2000 (http://www.mankato.msus.edu/dept/comdis/ISAD3/isadcon3.html):

The real world of jobs by Karen Lewis (Ohio, US), Gunars Neiders (Washington, US), Lee Reeves (Texas, US), Louis Roden (Georgia, US), David Steiner (New York, US), and Ann Van Der Berg (South Africa)

Intensive group therapy for 15 -18 year old young adults by Frances Cook and Jane Fry (United Kingdom)

Multicultural considerations in the treatment of stuttering by Fred Hall (Massachusetts, US)

Speech pathologists can help children who are teased because they stutter by Bill Murphy (Indiana, US)

The public environment where attitudes develop: Stuttering versus mental illness and intelligence by Kenneth O. St. Louis, James D. Schiffbauer, Carolyn I. Phillips, Andrea B. Sedlock, Lisa J. Hriblan, and Rebecca M. Dayton (West Virginia, US)

For the general public and new students of speech-language pathology with no background in stuttering

If you want to spend only 10 minutes...
Did you know...Fact sheet about stuttering. Memphis, TN: Stuttering Foundation of America. (Brochure: #47, www.stutteringhelp.org; 1-800-992-9392)

How to react when speaking with someone who stutters. Memphis, TN: Stuttering Foundation of America. (Brochure: #46, www.stutteringhelp.org; 1-800-992-9392, Spanish version: #63)

If you want to spend 30 minutes...
Do you stutter: Straight talk for teens. Memphis, TN: Stuttering Foundation of America. (Videotape: 30 minutes. www.stutteringhelp.org; 1-800-992-9392)

If you want to spend 2 hours...
St. Louis, K. O. (Ed.). (2001). *Living with Stuttering: Stories, Basics, Resources, and Hope.* Morgantown, WV: Populore Publishing Company. (1-866-667-8679)

If you want to spend 1 day, read/watch the above materials plus...

Browse Judy Kuster's "The Stuttering Homepage" http://www.stutteringhomepage.com

If you want to spend 5 days, read/watch the above materials plus...

Bondarenko, V. *Voices to remember* (Videotape: 60 minutes. US— Suncoast Media, 2938 West Bay Dr., Suite B, Belleair Bluffs, FL 34640; Canada—Magic Lantern Communications, 775 Pacific Road, Oakville, ONT L6L 6M4)

Browse through and read several articles from the 1st (1998), 2nd (1999), and 3rd (2000) International Stuttering Awareness Day (ISAD) On-Line Conferences. These were papers submitted electronically to "conferences" that began on October 1st each year and ended about three weeks later. During this period of each conference, individuals anywhere who had access to the World Wide Web were able to post questions or comments that could be answered or responded to by authors or other interested persons. Consider, especially, the following papers:

from 1998 (http://www.mankato.msus.edu/dept/comdis/isad/isadcon.html):

Adolescents who stutter: the urgent need for support groups (A parent's perspective), by Lee Caggiano (New York, US)

Consumer self-help and professional associations by Charlie Diggs (Maryland, US)

Some thoughts on the multidimensional nature of stuttering from a neurophysiological perspective by Luc De Nil (Toronto, Canada)

Issues of culture and stuttering: A South African perspective by Harsha Kathard (South Africa)

Internet resources about stuttering by Judith Kuster (Minnesota, US)

What is "successful" stuttering therapy? by Robert Quesal (Illinois, US)

The role of self-help/support groups in determining the outcomes of stuttering therapy by Lee Reeves (Texas, US)

A synopsis of cluttering and its treatment by Kenneth St. Louis (Virginia, US) and Florence Myers (New York, US)

Views from a wife by Harriet Weiner (Michigan, US)

from 1999 (http://www.mankato.msus.edu/dept/comdis/isad2/isadcon2.html):

Early intervention with childhood stuttering revisited by Richard F. Curlee (US)

The Hawthorne Effect and its impact on stuttering therapy by John Harrison (California, US)

Public speaking for stutterers by Russ Hicks (Texas, US)

Stuttering: The real world by Michael Hughes (Canada)

Creating your own map for change by Walter Manning (Tennessee, US)

Change by David Preece (United Kingdom)

"One size fits all (or: When the only tool you have is a hammer...)" by Bob Quesal (Illinois, US)

The stutterer's experience by C. Woodruff Starkweather (Pennsylvania, US)

The stereotyping of people who stutter: Origins, effects, and controls by Dale F. Williams & Carlos F. Diaz (Florida, US)

The Lidcombe Program: Where to next? by Michelle Lincoln (Australia)

The relationship between language and fluency in children and role of parents in managing stuttering by Nan Ratner (Maryland, US)

An animal model for stuttering-related part-word repetitions by David B. Rosenfield, Nagalapura S. Viswanath, Santosh A. Helekar. (Texas, US)

from 2000 (http://www.mankato.msus.edu/dept/comdis/ISAD3/isadcon3.html):

Children's books about stuttering, featuring Gail Wilson Lew (California US), Ellen-Marie Silverman (Wisconsin, US), Eelco de Geus (Netherlands), Ulrich Natke (Germany)

The real world of jobs by Karen Lewis (Ohio, US), Gunars Neiders (Washington, US), Lee Reeves (Texas, US), Louis Roden (Georgia, US), David Steiner (New York, US), and Ann Van Der Berg (South Africa)

Stuggling and juttering by Joe Donaher (Pennsylvania, US)

What parents can do for your child when he is being teased for stuttering by Gail Wilson Lew

Speech pathologists can help children who are teased because they stutter by Bill Murphy (Indiana, US)

Identification of stuttering in preschool children: A multifactorial longitudinal study in development by Hans Maansson (Denmark)

The public environment where attitudes develop: Stuttering versus mental illness and intelligence by Kenneth O. St. Louis, James D. Schiffbauer, Carolyn I. Phillips, Andrea B. Sedlock, Lisa J. Hriblan, and Rebecca M. Dayton (West Virginia, US)

Jezer, M. (1997). *Stuttering: A Life Bound up in Words.* New York: Basic Books.

For trained speech-language pathologists

...who either have had little training or clinical experience in stuttering therapy, who believe they need to update their information, or who wish to become Board Recognized Specialists in Fluency Disorders.

If you want to spend 2 hours...
St. Louis, K. O. (Ed.). (2001). *Living with Stuttering: Stories, Basics, Resources, and Hope.* Morgantown, WV: Populore Publishing Company. (1-866-667-8679)

If you want to spend 1 day, read the above book plus...
American Speech-Language-Hearing Association Special Interest Division 4: Fluency and Fluency Disorders. (1995, March). Guidelines for practice in stuttering treatment. *Asha, 37* (Suppl. 14), pp. 26-35

American Speech-Language-Hearing Association Special Interest Division 4: Fluency and Fluency Disorders. (1999, March). Terminology pertaining to fluency and fluency disorders: Guidelines. *Asha, 41* (Suppl. 19), pp. 29-36

Therapy in action: The school-age child who stutters. Memphis, TN: Stuttering Foundation of America. (Videotape: 38 minutes. www.stutteringhelp.org; 1-800-992-9392)

Do you stutter: Straight talk for teens. Memphis, TN: Stuttering Foundation of America. (Videotape: 30 minutes. www.stutteringhelp.org; 1-800-992-9392)

Browse Judy Kuster's "The Stuttering Homepage" http://www.stutteringhomepage.com

If you want to spend 5 days, read/watch the above materials plus…

Stuttering and your child: A videotape for parents. Memphis, TN: Stuttering Foundation of America. (Videotape: 30 minutes. www.stutteringhelp.org; 1-800-992-9392)

If you stutter: Advice for adults. Memphis, TN: Stuttering Foundation of America. (Videotape: 60 minutes. www.stutteringhelp.org; 1-800-992-9392)

Bondarenko, V. *Voices to remember* (Videotape: 60 minutes. US—Suncoast Media, 2938 West Bay Dr. Suite B, Belleair Bluffs, FL 34640; Canada—Magic Lantern Communications, 775 Pacific Road, Oakville, ONT L6L 6M4)

Guitar, B. (1998). *Stuttering: An Integrated Approach to its Nature and Treatment* (2nd Ed.). (www.wwilkins.com; 1-800-638-0672)

If you want to spend 1 to 2 months on some evenings and weekends, read/watch the above materials plus…

Choose one of these three:

Conture, E. G. (2001). *Stuttering: Its Nature, Diagnosis, and Treatment* (3rd Ed.). Boston: Allyn & Bacon. (www.abacon.com; 1-800-278-3525)

Manning, W. H. (2001). *Clinical Decision Making in Fluency Disorders* (2nd Ed.). San Diego, CA: Singular. (www.singpub.com; 1-800-842-3636)

Shapiro, D. A. (1999). *Stuttering intervention: A Collaborative Journey to Fluency Freedom*. Austin, TX: Pro-Ed. (www.proedinc.com; 1-800-897-3202)

Choose two of these three:

Bloodstein, O. (1995). *A Handbook on Stuttering* (5th Ed.). San Diego, CA: Singular. (www.singpub.com; 1-800-842-3636)

Curlee, R. F. (Ed.). (1999). *Stuttering and Related Disorders of Fluency* (2nd Ed.). New York: Thieme. (www.thieme.com; 1-800-782-3488)

Curlee, R. F. & Siegel, G. M. (Eds.). (1997). *Nature and Treatment of Stuttering: New Directions* (2nd Ed.). Needham Heights, MA: Allyn & Bacon. (www.abacon.com; 1-800-278-3525)

If you want to become a Board Recognized Specialist in Fluency Disorders to treat stuttering and other fluency disorders...

Contact the Specialty Board on Fluency Disorders to 1) Obtain a list of Board Recognized Mentors, 2) Contact, interview, and select a mentor who is willing to help you through the process of becoming a specialist, 3) Negotiate the fee (if any) that your mentor will charge for his or her services, 4) Prepare a plan with your mentor and submit it for approval by the Specialty Board on Fluency Disorders, 5) Under the direction and supervision of your mentor (and other designated clinicians), carry out the necessary coursework, continuing education, and guided practice with at least three fluency disordered individuals representing different age and severity levels and different approaches to therapy, 6) In consultation with your mentor, prepare a portfolio for approval by the Specialty Board for Fluency Disorders, 7) Take and pass the Specialty Board on Fluency Disorders written examination, and 8) Pay any necessary fees.

Contact Information: Specialty Board on Fluency Disorders; Current Address: Memphis Speech and Hearing Center,

807 Jefferson Avenue, Memphis, TN 38105. Or, contact the Division Coordinator in charge of the Special Interest Division 4 on Fluency and Fluency Disorders of the American Speech-Language-Hearing Association (http://professional.asha.org/sidivisions/sid_4.htm; 1-800-498-2071) for the Board's address or website.

As part of becoming a specialist, you may wish to attend a therapy program as an observer or clinician. Alternatively, you may apply to attend a week-long workshop on stuttering therapy at Northwestern University or in other sites around the country co-sponsored by the Stuttering Foundation of America.

Contact Information: Jane Fraser, Stuttering Foundation of America, 3100 Walnut Grove Road, Suite 603, PO Box 11749, Memphis, TN 38111-0749; www.stutteringhelp.org; 1-800-992-9392.

Taking Stock

Before deciding to seek help with your stuttering, perhaps for the first time or again if you had speech therapy as a child, I suggest that you carry out a self-study exercise that I call "taking stock." I wrote about taking stock as an early step of therapy in Chapter 26 called "Your Life is Too Important to Spend It Worrying About Stuttering," in The Stuttering Foundation of America publication #9, *Advice to Those Who Stutter*.

In this book I have provided two activities that may help you do that. First, consider telling your own story of stuttering, somewhat like the various authors in *Chapter 2: Our Stories*. *Appendix G: Taking Stock: Telling Your Story* provides some helpful guidelines on how to do that, even if none of your friends or family ever sees or hears the story (though it would be very helpful for your future speech-language pathologist). The second thing you might do is go to *Appendix H: Taking Stock: Assessing Your Life Perspectives and Stuttering* which explains the *St. Louis Inventory of Life Perspectives and Stuttering (SL•ILP-S)*. You might find it helpful to fill out an *SL•ILP-S* for the present time, and an *SL•ILP-S/R* both for when you were about ten years old and when you were in high school to see what changes might have occurred over time.

Locating Resources

In the same *Advice to Those Who Stutter* chapter mentioned above, I also recommended "locating resources." This is an important, but sometimes difficult, step. It is normal when learning something new to be overwhelmed with the amount of confusing and contradictory information we have to sift through. The same is true of seeking resources for stuttering therapy.

Therapy, self-help, or both?

This book, *Living with Stuttering: Stories, Basics, Resources, and Hope*, especially the information in the appendices, is specifically designed to help you understand important options you have at your disposal. The first decision you must make is whether you prefer to seek speech therapy, assistance from a self-help group, or both. If you decide you do not want, do not have the financial resources for, or do not have access to speech therapy, then you might want to skip the following sections on speech therapy and go directly to the section on self-help resources.

Qualifications of speech-language pathologists

If you are seeking speech therapy, ideally you will find a speech-language pathologist who has the interest and expertise to help you. Let me review some facts about speech-language pathologists' qualifications. First, be aware that in the US, most of the states (46) have licensure laws that govern the practice of speech-language pathology (http://professional.asha.org/membership/licensure.htm). However, we must deal with two important facts. States vary in the necessary academic requirements to qualify for licensure. And, speech-language pathologists in the public schools do not need to be licensed because school personnel—like teachers—are required only to meet certification standards developed by state Boards of Education. The best assurance of minimum qualifications in fluency disorders—although this is no guarantee of expertise—is the Certificate of Clinical Competence in Speech-Language Pathology (typically abbreviated CCC/SLP) from the American Speech-Language-Hearing Association (ASHA). Individuals with "their Cs" must have graduated with at least a master's degree that required more than 300 hours of supervised clinical practicum and have completed a year of work under the general supervision of a certified individual (known as the Clinical Fellowship Year). (In Canada, the equivalent certification is from the Canadian Association of Speech-Language Pathologists and Audiologists.) There are a sizable number of practicing speech-language pathologists, especially in the public school systems of some states, who do not hold master's degrees.

Locating Board Recognized Specialists in Fluency Disorders

If possible, try to seek out a speech-language pathologist who has the CCC/SLP. However, considerable amount of survey research has shown that you cannot assume that everyone with "Cs" feels comfortable working with stuttering; in fact, a majority prefer not to do so. Where do you turn? As I noted before, there is a new specialty recognition program that was recently developed by the Special Interest Division 4 on Fluency and Fluency Disorders of ASHA. The new Specialty Board on Fluency Disorders, a separate professional entity which voluntarily collaborates with ASHA, recognized about 300 new specialists in fluency disorders in 2000 and 2001. These individuals are certified by ASHA, have at least five years of professional experience, and are well trained and experienced in treating people who stutter. They are committed to a regular process of continuing education in fluency disorders and must renew their specialty status every three years. In addition, the Specialty Board is just beginning a training and mentoring program designed to help interested but less experienced ASHA certified speech-language pathologists become specialists in fluency disorders. Three hundred specialists in fluency disorders is a minuscule percentage of ASHA's nearly 100,000 members. But it's a start. The program is so new that there is not yet a website or clearinghouse indicating the names and locations of Board Recognized Specialists in Fluency Disorders, but that will soon occur. You can find out who is on that list by contacting: the Specialty Board on Fluency Disorders, Memphis Speech and Hearing Center, 807 Jefferson Avenue, Memphis, TN 38105 or by contacting ASHA (http://professional.asha.org/sidivisions/sid_4.htm; 1-800-498-2071) for the Board's current address or website.

Locating clinicians who have expressed
interest in treating stuttering

It is likely that there might not be a specialist in your area. The next best place to check is the Stuttering Foundation of America (SFA) Referral List (www.stutteringhelp.org; 1-800-992-9392). The SFA publishes a list of over 400 speech-language pathologists in the USA on their website and updates it each year. The web page is arranged by state, and by clicking on your state, you can find speech-language pathologists who have indicated that they are interested in and are competent to treat stuttering. (The SFA can neither guarantee the competence of these clinicians nor make any implications about speech-language pathologists who are not on the list.) In the future, it is likely that the list will also indicate who is a Board Recognized Specialist. It should be noted that the SFA also has a listing of professionals in other countries who wish to be listed as referral sources for stuttering.

If you contact a person on either of the above lists who cannot help you, perhaps because of time or distance, ask if he or she can refer you, directly or through another person, to someone in your area who has special expertise, experience, or interest in stuttering.

Discussing your needs and wants with potential clinicians

As you locate and interview potential clinicians, you might want to ask them about their philosophy of stuttering treatment and how they proceed with individuals such as you. Most competent clinicians are readily willing and able to discuss this. In fact, ASHA's Code of Ethics, to which certified speech-language pathologists are bound, "shall fully inform the persons they serve of the nature and possible effects of services rendered and products dispensed" and "shall not…misrepresent, in any fashion, services rendered or products dispensed." This does not mean that you should expect any kind of guarantee. Guarantees are not possible and, in fact, the code of ethics forbids making them.

My advice would be to listen to the clinician about what he or she thinks is your best course of treatment. Many times, there is no "best" approach; several could be effective. If you do have a strong preference for fluency shaping, for example, feel free to mention it. If you have worked very hard at fluency shaping in the past and not found it particularly helpful and, as a result, want to try stuttering modification, mention that as well. Obviously, you don't typically tell your doctor how to treat you! So remembering that while the clinician needs to ultimately decide the direction of therapy, a frank, joint conversation about the cost, direction, duration, and possible outcomes of treatment with a new clinician is often a positive experience for all parties involved. If you want more information about various therapies for stuttering and programs that provide them, click on "Therapy for Stuttering" on Judy Kuster's The Stuttering Homepage to get a comprehensive listing (www.stutteringhomepage.com).

Intensive stuttering therapy programs

You may wish to attend an intensive therapy program to become fluent. If so, The Stuttering Homepage has such information. So does the SFA website, which lists both year-round and summer intensive programs in the US and Canada, each followed by contact information and a description of the program and costs (www.stutteringhelp.org; 1-800-992-9392). ASHA has a fairly comprehensive listing of summer therapy programs, although descriptions are not provided (http://professional.asha.org/consumers/camps/camp_fluency.htm;1-800-498-2071). Remember that in many of these intensive programs, you will not have the flexibility to "write your own program" although individual needs are always addressed. Typically, you go through the therapy program as part of a group.

Following is a sampling of programs from the above lists that are well known, widely respected, and appropriate for adolescents or adults who stutter. I cannot overemphasize the point that omission from this list should not be construed to reflect negatively on omitted programs.

The American Institute for Stuttering
www.stutteringtreatment.org; 877-378-8883; Catherine Otto Montgomery, 27 West 20th Street, Suite 1203, New York, NY 10011; AIS@stutteringtreatment.org.

The Annandale Fluency Clinic, Inc.
www.afccafet.com; 703-941-8903; Martha Goebel, 4208 Evergreen Lane, Suite 213, Annandale, VA 22003; mgoebel@afccafet.com.

Birch Tree Foundation
215-222-4559; C. Woodruff (Woody) Starkweather, 3615 Hamilton Street, Philadelphia, PA 19104; v5002e@vm.temple.edu.

Boston University, Department of Communication Disorders
617-353-4778; Adriana Digrande, Boston University, Department of Communication Disorders, 635 Commonwealth Avenue, Boston, MA 02115; digrande@bu.edu.

Columbia Speech and Language Services
604-875-9100; #1316 - 750 W Broadway, Vancouver, BC V5Z 1J3, Canada; speech@interchange.ubc.ca.

Comprehensive Stuttering Program
www.ualberta.ca/~istar/; 780-492-2619; Deborah Kully-Martens, The Institute for Stuttering Treatment and Research, 3rd Floor, Aberhart

Centre Two, 8220 - 114 Street, Edmonton, Alberta T6G 2P4, Canada; istar@gpu.srv.ualberta.ca.

Fluency Intensive Center for Communication Disorders
212-481-4464; Dorothy Ross, Hunter College, 425 East 25th Street, New York, NY 10010; dorothyross@hunter.cuny.edu.

Harold B. Starbuck Memorial Fluency Enhancing Clinics
www.geneseo.edu; 716-245-5328; Kathleen R. Jones, Department of Communicative Disorders and Sciences, State University of New York at Geneseo, Geneseo, NY 14454-1401; jonesk@uno.cc.geneseo.edu. (Note: programs are run in both Geneseo, NY, and Ben Lomond, CA.)

Hollins Fluency System
www.stuttering.org; 540-265-5650; Ronald Webster, Hollins Communications Research, PO Box 9737, Roanoke, VA 24020; adm-heri@rbnet.com.

Indiana University/Sertoma Speech Camp For Teens Who Stutter
www.indiana.edu/~bradwood; 812-855-3664; Ann Densmore, Indiana University Department of Speech and Hearing Sciences, 200 S. Jordan Avenue, Bloomington, IN 47405; adensmor@indiana.edu.

Pennsylvania State University
814-865-3177; Gordon Blood, Department of Communication Disorders, 110 Moore Building. University Park, PA 16802.

Power Stuttering Center
714-427-0477; Mark Power, Intensive Stutter Free Speech Program, 2775 Mesa Verde Drive East, #T 202, Costa Mesa, CA 92626; jmpower@ix.netcom.com.

Precision Fluency Shaping Program
757-446-5938; Ross Barrett, Eastern Virginia Medical School, 825 Fairfax Avenue, Norfolk, VA 23507; pfsp@aol.com.

Speech Foundation of Ontario
416-323-3335; Robert Kroll, Stuttering Centre, 5 Sultan Street, Toronto, Ontario M5S 1L6, Canada; bob.kroll@utoronto.ca.

Successful Stuttering Management Program (two sites)
509-359-2302; Kim Krieger, Department of Communication Disorders, MS-106, Eastern Washington University, 526 5th Street, Cheney, WA 99004-2431.

801-293-8400; Tom Gurrister, University of Utah, Department of Communication Disorders, 1201 Behavioral Sciences Building, Salt Lake City, UT 84112; tgurrister@aol.com.

Summer Remedial Clinic
517-774-3472; Colin McPherson, Central Michigan University, Moore Hall, 444, Mt. Pleasant, MI 48859; colin.a.macpherson@cmich.edu.

Wendell Johnson Speech and Hearing Clinic
Intensive Stuttering Program For Teens
319-335-8735 or 319-335-8744; Patricia M. Zebrowski or Toni D. Cilek, Wendell Johnson Speech and Hearing Clinic, Hawkins Drive, University of Iowa, Iowa City, IA 52242-1012; tricia-zebrowski@uiowa.edu or toni_cilek@uiowa.edu.

Self-help groups for people who stutter

Whether or not you choose to attend speech therapy, you may wish to participate in or even start a stuttering self-help or support group.

The Stuttering Homepage
The Stuttering Homepage is an excellent source for information about self-help or support groups. Click on "Support Organizations for PWS" to see a comprehensive listing of support groups around the world (www.stutteringhomepage.com).

The National Stuttering Association (NSA)
The National Stuttering Association, formerly the National Stuttering Project, is the largest self-help group for people who stutter in the US. It has more than seventy-five chapters nationwide and serves more than 2700 members. The NSA develops and promotes information for people who stutter, publishes a newsletter called *Letting Go,* and has an annual convention. It recently began providing continuing education opportunities for speech-language pathologists. Contact information: www.nsastutter.org; 1-800-364-1677; 5100 East La Palma, Suite #208, Anaheim Hills, CA 92807.

Friends
Friends is a relatively new organization for young people who stutter and their parents. Friends also hosts an annual convention and publishes a newsletter called *Reaching Out.* Contact Information: www.friendswhostutter.org; John Ahlbach, 1220 Rosita Road, Pacifica, CA 94044-4223.

Canadian Association for People Who Stutter (CAPS)
The Canadian Association for People Who Stutter is a national non-profit organization that provides coordination for a national network of autonomous Canadian self-help groups for people who stutter. This umbrella organization has a newsletter called *CAPS News,* and it, too,

sponsors regular conferences. Contact information: www.webcon.net/~caps/; 1-888-788-8837; CAPS, PO Box 444, Succ. N.D.G., Montreal QC H4A 3P8, Canada.

Speak Easy Inc. of Canada
www.speakeasycanada.com; Speak Easy of Canada, similar to Speak Easy organizations in the US and other countries, provides information and support to adult stutterers, parents of stuttering children, professionals in the field, and the general public. It has a newsletter entitled, *Speaking Out.*

International Stuttering Association (ISA)
http://www.semico.org/stutter-2001; The International Stuttering Association is an umbrella organization of self-help and support groups around the world. The ISA publishes a newsletter called *One Voice* and hosts international congresses for people who stutter.

Professional organizations that deal with stuttering

American Speech-Language-Hearing Association (ASHA)
http://professional.asha.org; 1-800-498-2071; ASHA is the major professional organization of nearly 100,000 speech-language pathologists and audiologists in the US. It represents the interests of members engaged in a wide variety of professional activities. Fluency disorders (which includes stuttering) is just one of the speech, language, or hearing disorders categories that ASHA members study and treat. ASHA sends its members a newspaper-like biweekly publication called *The ASHA Leader.* There is also a quarterly magazine-styled journal called *Asha.* ASHA also publishes four professional journals, three of which regularly carry articles on stuttering: the *American Journal of Speech-Language Pathology*; *Language, Speech, and Hearing Services in Schools*; and the *Journal of Speech, Language, and Hearing Research.* In addition, ASHA has a great many other resources available for its members, consumers such as people who stutter, and the public. The annual convention of ASHA typically draws 10,000 to 12,000 members.

Special Interest Division 4 on Fluency and Fluency Disorders (SID 4)
http://professional.asha.org/sidivisions/sid_4.htm; In the past decade, ASHA members have been able to join 15 different Special Interest Divisions (SIDs) as well. SID 4 is the one related to stuttering and, in 2001, had approximately 800 members. SID 4 is run by an elected Steering Committee from the membership and has a quarterly newsletter that deals with issues of concern to those of us who work in the area of fluency disorders. SID 4 hosts an annual leadership conference devoted to selected topics.

Specialty Board on Fluency Disorders
(Website under development) The Specialty Board on Fluency Disorders is a new, independent body consisting of five members who are elected to three-year terms by the SID 4 membership. The Board's mission is to inaugurate, oversee, and maintain a program of Board Recognized Specialists in Fluency Disorders. It interfaces with ASHA voluntarily through ASHA's Council on Clinical Specialty Recognition. Currently there are more than 300 specialists in the inaugural cadre of specialists. A group of mentors in fluency disorders is being developed to work with new applicants to go through a carefully supervised process of becoming recognized specialists. Specialists in fluency disorders must be renewed every three years, and mentors undergo renewal every five years.

**Canadian Association of Speech-Language Pathologists
and Audiologists (CASLPA)**
www.caslpa.ca; 1-800-259-8519; This is the professional association in Canada that parallels ASHA in the US. Like ASHA members, CASLPA members deal with a wide array of speech, language, and hearing disorders. Certified members of CASLPA are eligible to be certified by ASHA, and vice versa, as a result of a reciprocity agreement between the two associations. It publishes the *Journal of Speech-Language Pathology and Audiology* and a quarterly member bulletin, *Communiqué*.

**US and Canadian state, provincial, and regional
speech, language, and hearing associations**
Most of the states in the US and provinces of Canada have their own speech-language pathology and audiology professional associations. Most of these associations have newsletters and annual conventions or meetings with their respective states, provinces, or regions. The US state associations can be accessed either through ASHA, clicking on "Certification and Membership" and then individual states (http://professional.asha.org/membership/licensure.htm) or via the Council of State Association Presidents of the American-Speech-Language-Hearing Association website (www.csap.org/who/stofficers.htm). Canadian associations can be reached through the CASLPA website (www.caslpa.ca/english/contacts/province2.htm).

International Association of Logopedics and Phoniatrics (IALP)
www1.ldc.lu.se/logopedi/IALP/sid1.html; IALP is an international association of professionals who deal with speech, language, voice, swallowing, and hearing disorders. The organization has two major subfields (logopedics and phoniatrics) that are based on a European model. It has nearly 500 individual members and fifty-six affiliated national societies from more than fifty countries. It publishes *Folia Phoniatrica et Logopedica*. The IALP has an international congress every three years.

International Fluency Association (IFA)
http://www.ruhr-uni-bochum.de/ifa/index.html; The International Fluency Association is an interdisciplinary, worldwide organization of clinicians, researchers, and people who stutter. Currently the IFA has about 300 members from thirty countries. It publishes the only international professional journal related entirely to fluency disorders, the *Journal of Fluency Disorders*. The IFA sponsors a world congress on fluency disorders every three years.

Information resources and clearinghouses on stuttering

Stuttering Foundation of America (SFA)
www.stutteringhelp.org; 1-800-992-9392; The Stuttering Foundation of America, formerly known as the Speech Foundation of America, is no doubt the world's leading resource for printed material designed for people who stutter and the general public. The SFA was founded more than fifty years ago by the late Malcolm Fraser and is now run by his daughter, Jane Fraser. The SFA has a wide variety of brochures, posters, books, and videotapes that are made available to anyone who orders them at a very reasonable cost. (Libraries can receive materials without cost upon request for specific materials.) It also sponsors and supports training workshops for speech-language pathologists and a few carefully chosen research projects.

The Stuttering Homepage
www.stutteringhomepage.com; Judy Kuster at Minnesota State University at Mankato has developed a website that has quickly become one of the best resources available for the public and people who stutter. Updated frequently, it provides solid information related to fluency disorders (e.g., stuttering and cluttering), listings of therapy articles and providers, and numerous other issues of interest to persons who stutter, the general public, and speech-language pathologists.

Interactive electronic lists

STUT-HLP
This list was founded and is owned by Bob Quesal, an author in this book. STUT-HLP is an open list in which stutterers and others can interact on-line in a supportive way. To subscribe: Send an email message to: lisproc2@ecnet.net. Type "subscribe Stut-hlp yourfirstname yourlastname" in the body of the message and send.

STUTT-X

Don Mowrer owns this open list, which is intended for discussions of stuttering and other speech-language disorders. To subscribe: Send an email message to: listserv@asuvm.inre.asu.edu. Type "subscribe Stutt-x yourfirstname yourlastname" in the body of the message and send.

STUTT-L

This list, started by Woody Starkweather, is intended for researchers and clinicians who work with stuttering. It now includes people who stutter as well. To subscribe: Send an email message to: listserv@vm.temple.edu. Type "subscribe Stutt-l yourfirstname yourlastname" in the body of the message and send.

International Stuttering Awareness Day (ISAD)

On-Line Conference threaded discussions. Since 1998, each year on October 22, the International Stuttering Awareness Day (ISAD) On-Line Conference begins. During the duration of the conference (a period of about three weeks), anyone can pose questions or post answers or comments to papers that are included in the conferences in the "threaded discussion" following each paper or topic. The ISAD conference can be reached through The Stuttering Homepage (www.stutteringhomepage.com), which also archives past conferences.

APPENDIX D: BILL OF RIGHTS AND RESPONSIBILITIES FOR PEOPLE WHO STUTTER

Preamble

Established in 2000, the Bill of Rights and Responsibilities for People who Stutter is a joint project by people who stutter, professional clinicians, and researchers. It provides a framework for building a more humane, just, and compassionate world for the millions of people who stutter.

In our society, speech is considered one of the most important means for interpersonal communication. While other means, such as written language, may be superior at times in conveying the content of messages, spoken language not only contains the content, but also includes information about the speaker's intent, emotions, personality, and perceptions. That is why people who read books still like to attend readings by authors of these books, and why millions of dollars are being spent developing tools that allow for automatic voice recognition systems and the incorporation of voice and images in electronic communication.

Unfortunately, the window speech provides on the speaker's self also can lead to stereotypical perceptions of people with speech disorders that go well beyond their speech difficulties.

While spoken word is taken for granted by most, the use of spoken language is challenging for millions of people who stutter around the world. It is estimated that approximately 1%, or 60 million, of the 6 billion people with whom we share this world stutter. For many of these individuals, daily communication is a constant struggle. For many of them, speech does not open doors but closes them for interpersonal, academic and professional development and fulfillment. Despite advances in our understanding of stuttering and its treatment, many people who stutter around the world do not have access to the services and support they deserve.

This Bill is written to foster attitudes and actions whereby individuals who stutter are provided the opportunity to fulfill their aspirations and to lead successful, productive lives. It recognizes the dual responsibility of listeners and society to create the environment in which people who stutter can develop their aspirations and talents, and of people who stutter to advocate better understanding and to become active partners in their own future.

Note:

The initial draft of this document was prepared by participants at the International Stuttering Awareness Day "Bill of Rights Workshop" facilitated by Michael Sugarman and Amy Johnson at the 17th Convention of the National Stuttering Association in Chicago, Illinois, in July 2000. That draft was modified based on feedback from participants at the International Fluency Association Third World Congress in Nyborg, Denmark, in August 2000. A new draft was circulated in January 2001 and, based on feedback, became this latest version to be ratified by various stuttering associations.

People who stutter have a right to...

Stutter or to be fluent to the extent one is able or chooses;

Communicate and be listened to regardless of one's degree of stuttering;

Be treated with dignity and respect by individuals, groups, institutions, and the media;

Publicly available and accurate information about stuttering;

Equal protection under the law regardless of one's degree of stuttering;

Be informed fully about therapy programs, including the likelihood of success, failure, or relapse;

Receive therapy appropriate for one's unique needs, concerns, and characteristics from professionals trained to treat stuttering and its related problems; and

Choose and participate in therapy, to choose not to do so, or to change therapy or clinician without prejudice or penalty.

People who stutter have a responsibility to...

Understand that listeners or conversation partners may be uninformed about stuttering and its ramifications or that they may hold different views of stuttering;

Advise listeners or conversation partners if one needs additional time to communicate;

Participate voluntarily in therapy in an open, active and cooperative manner;

Do whatever one can to overcome life handicaps that have occurred because of stuttering. This includes developing a realistic appraisal of one's strengths and weaknesses;

Regard and treat others who have problems, disabilities, or handicaps with fairness under the law and with dignity and respect, regardless of the nature of their conditions; and

Educate the public about stuttering and its ramifications.

I cannot convey all I have learned about people who stutter during the compilation of this book, and I can never fully express the gratitude that I have for the stutterers who chose to share their own stories and reveal the emotions, attitudes, and triumphs that make up their lives as stutterers. Their courage has enabled me to realize the power of the stutterer's story as a therapy tool, not only to build trust with my clients and provide a starting point for therapy, but also to round and refine myself as a person and clinician through the experiences of others.

Stories can teach...

The difficulties presented to people in life are not to be taken at face value; instead, therapy outcomes may greatly depend on the person's perception of the problem and his or her strength, creativity, and desire to overcome it. As a student and a future speech-language pathologist, I believe this is one of the most important things to realize before diving in elbow deep to help solve or change a client's problem.

Crystal Hightower, senior honor student majoring in speech pathology, with her cousin Autumn.

While reading interview transcripts for more than 100 stutterers for this project, I realized that this rings especially true for the stuttering population. I have found that people who stutter as a whole are intelligent, thoughtful, and sensitive people coming from all walks of life. They experience the same joys as well as the same pain as the people who surround them and walk beside them in life. But, they also carry the burden of a speech difficulty that affects them in their own personal way and that is highly individualized and sometimes very emotional. The stories in this book show how stuttering may interfere with a person's social life, academic life, or career choices. And they show how it can regulate perceptions as well as fears or joys, but also how, for some, it can have little or no effect at all.

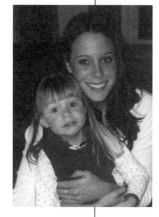

As I read them, I was able to understand the diversity of the population, but I also saw many of the universalities of the emotions revealed in the words. I've learned that it is necessary to relate to the person and his or her experiences and emotions before beginning therapy. In fact, many stutterers decide that therapy is not the best option for them because of past negative experiences, which only makes my job as a clinician more difficult. I would prefer to know the most difficult situations in their lives along with the easiest, the ways that stuttering has affected their choices in life, and the way that they have dealt with their problem and others' reactions to it.

With this knowledge, I would know where to begin, the sensitivities of the client, and the basis from which to build rapport. By asking stutterers to tell their stories, I can gain much of this information, begin to win their trust, and construct a therapy plan that will hopefully create a positive experience.

Using this book...

Using the forms and worksheets described in this book, I could give my own clients a starting point from which to begin their stories. I may then learn how stuttering has affected their lives, how they have dealt with it, the positives and negatives that they perceive from their experiences as stutterers, and most importantly, their goals and aspirations.

After obtaining information about the development of their problem (along with its exacerbations and remissions) and future goals, I as a professional could choose a therapy plan that fits the client as a person. Many of the currently accepted therapy techniques and approaches are outlined in this book. Also presented are the positives and negatives associated with each approach. This book's author holds a unique and trustworthy viewpoint as not only an experienced clinician with a specialty in stuttering, but also as a stutterer himself. Whether you are a clinician in the making, a practicing clinician in need of more information, or a stutterer seeking self-education, you can read through the outlined techniques and choose a starting point appropriate for your client or yourself.

Many parts of this book would also be helpful as an information source for stutterers. For example, stutterers can find comfort in knowing that they are not alone in their struggles with communication. They may seek this comfort by reading and learning from the lives of others with the same problem, and they may find consolation and encouragement in relating to many of the same experiences, fears, triumphs, and emotions expressed in the stories of these stutterers' lives.

Like our clients and their families, we, as clinicians, may benefit from a concrete definition of the struggles or descriptions of the therapy techniques we can choose for them. The book contains fast facts, easy definitions, and experiences that provide such information. Finally, if the client requires information beyond our knowledge, they can consult the references and contact sources.

Most courses in stuttering focus on facts, figures, and techniques. Of course, we expect the tried and true techniques to work when we are faced with a stuttering client, but much more is required. Many of the "constants" in stuttering are often uniquely influenced by a person's experiences, perceptions of stuttering, and the reactions of other people. Stuttering therapy must strive to touch each and every one of these experiences, to replace negative emotions and attitudes with positive ones, and to find the best techniques to modify the stuttering. After this is set into motion, it is more likely that the client will begin the process of developing a healthier attitude, taking charge of his or her own goals, and accepting responsibility for the outcomes of experiences with stuttering.

Interviewing can be a powerful learning experience...

The majority of the stories presented in *Chapter 2: Our Stories* were prepared from interviews conducted by speech pathology students. Among these student interviewers, the consensus of opinion seems to be that the interview process was extremely worthwhile and, in many cases, quite eye-opening:

"I really learned a lot from the interview and I may never experience the embarrassment, but I feel as though I can now have empathy for a client who has a stuttering disorder."

"I learned from this experience to be a great listener. Listening is an important part of being a speech pathologist, and shows that the clinician cares for the well-being of his/her client."

"I realized that there are many things I do each day without thinking that are very difficult for a person who stutters."

"I learned that a positive attitude can get you through life and enable you to do many things, regardless of the limitations placed upon you."

"I asked him whether it is better to be called a 'stutterer' or a 'person who stutters.' His reply was 'Neither—I am just a person; everyone has their flaws.'"

"I learned that stutterers are judged by the way they speak before it is found out who they really are."

"I learned that a healthy sense of humor can be a great benefit to someone with a speech problem."

"I think I learned that it's really true when they say you need to be able to treat the whole person and not just the disorder."

Many students take only one undergraduate course in stuttering, and if they are lucky, an additional course in graduate school. Direct access to stutterers' experiences may or may not be available to them. Because of this lack of exposure, a beginning clinician may not know where to begin with a stuttering client. Many times I have heard students say that they lack the confidence necessary to counsel and provide therapy for a person who stutters. Much of this lack of confidence stems from a reluctance to deal with an awkward communication situation. As I helped with the preparation of this book, I was able to confront and release some of my own fears of working with the stuttering population. After learning about the experiences of stutterers, their clinicians, and their struggles (or lack thereof), I feel comfortable looking past their communication problem to see the stutterer as a person with experiences to share and stories to tell.

Author: Crystal D. Hightower.

Crystal received her bachelor's degree from West Virginia University in May 2001 in Speech Pathology and Audiology. She is currently continuing her graduate studies there. As part of an independent research project, she assisted the author with this book project. Her key contribution was as Story Editor. Crystal spends her spare time at the gym or doing outdoor activities with her parents and her boyfriend, Justin. She hopes to return to her home town, Beckley, West Virginia, to practice as a certified speech-language pathologist.

AMERICAN
SPEECH-LANGUAGE-
HEARING
ASSOCIATION

Terminology Pertaining to Fluency and Fluency Disorders: Guidelines

ASHA Special Interest Division 4: Fluency and Fluency Disorders

These guidelines are an official statement of the American Speech-Language-Hearing Association (ASHA). They provide guidance on definitions of communication disorders and variations, but are not official standards of the Association. They were developed by Special Interest Division 4, Fluency and Fluency Disorders: Gordon W. Blood, Hugo H. Gregory, John M. Hanley, Stephen B. Hood, Theodore J. Peters, Kenneth O. St. Louis (chair), C. Woodruff Starkweather, and Janice B. Westbrook. Vice Presidents for Professional Practices in Speech-Language Pathology, Crystal Cooper (1994–1996), and Nancy Creaghead (1997–1999), served as monitoring vice presidents; Lyn Goldberg and Michelle Ferketic were ex officios.

1. Introduction

The *fluency* area is plagued with inconsistent, confusing terminology. This problem has cultural, historical, linguistic, and practical origins. The following examples illustrate some of these influences. In most cultures, *stuttering* is one of the most well-known speech disorders and is labeled in some form in all languages. In some languages, the label is a relatively neutral, descriptive term that refers to both normal and abnormal behavior. In English, for example, *stuttering* can refer to normal stumbling over words or to the abnormal speech disorder. This leaves English speakers confused about the best meaning of the term and contributes to one of the most difficult issues in definition, notably that most normal speak-

Reference this material as: American Speech-Language-Hearing Association Special Interest Division 4: Fluency and Fluency Disorders. (1999, March). Terminology pertaining to fluency and fluency disorders: Guidelines. *Asha, 41* (Suppl. 19), 29–36.

Index terms: accessory (secondary) behaviors, cluttering, definitions, disfluency, dysfluency, effort, fluency, fluency disorder, naturalness, neurogenic stuttering, prosody, psychogenic stuttering, rate, rhythm, suprasegmental features, stutterer, stuttering, terminology

ing adults report that they have "*stuttered*" occasionally but emphatically do not regard themselves as "*stutterers.*" (The issue of using the direct label, *stutterer*, versus the person-first label, person who *stutters*, is discussed in section 3.5.5.) Yet, even when it is clear that abnormal speech is implied, *stuttering* may also refer to a general style of speech (i.e., "That person *stutters*") or to specific speech events (i.e., "His primary *stuttering* symptom is part-word repetitions"). In other languages, such as Arabic, the terms for *stuttering* carry serious negative connotations and refer not only to a speech disorder but to other problems, such as mental incapacity. Furthermore, society often forms perceptions of individuals who *stutter* that differ from the self-perceptions of the *stutterers* themselves. Added to these problems is the fact that the literature on speech and language disorders contains terminology introduced in early classifications but rarely used today (e.g., a semantic distinction between *stuttering* and *stammering*).

2. Intent and Use of the Guidelines

The problem of terminology has been most acute in the area of research, in which defensible, reliable, and agreed-on definitions are critical to carrying out investigations that are comparable to other studies. Clinicians, too, need to know what constitutes *stuttering* and other *fluency disorders* in order to plan treatment and to communicate effectively with their clients and other clinicians. Additionally, the demands of health care systems require that providers strive for consistency and clarity of terminology, especially in reporting assessment and outcome measures. For these reasons, the terms highlighted in these Guidelines are defined with the intention that more consistent usage and, thereby, more precise communication by researchers, clinicians, and others will eventually result. Whenever possible, the Task Force sought to recommend terminology and definitions currently being utilized by well-known professionals. Clinicians, health care professionals, and researchers are encouraged to use the terms in bold type whenever possible. In some cases, the definitions listed can be used accurately in most contexts. In other cases, however, users are cautioned to keep the purposes of their definitions in mind. For example, there are four different definitions of the term *stuttering*, each representing important aspects of the problem and unique perspectives on definition. It would be a serious mistake for a user to select any one of the *stuttering* definitions and assume that it would apply equally well for teaching, clinical, research, consumer affairs, and third-party reimbursement purposes. For each term, the definitions the Task Force considered to be the preferred usage are in bold type. These are followed by relevant explanations or brief discussions and, in some cases, synonymous—or nearly synonymous—terms.

3. Definitions and Comments

3.1. Fluency. Fluency is the aspect of speech production that refers to the continuity, smoothness, rate, and/or effort with which phonologic, lexical, morphologic, and/or syntactic language units are spoken.

Traditionally, fluency has been defined in the area of speech-language pathology by what it is not, namely speech that does not contain perceptible deviations in smoothness or flow of speech. Also, in a more restricted clinical sense, *fluency* is used as the converse of *stuttering* to identify speech sequences that are free of *stuttering*, as in the statement, "*Stuttering* was followed by instructions to repeat, and *fluency* was reinforced verbally." And in recent years, *fluency* has been used increasingly to refer specifically to *stuttering* (e.g., "a *fluency* client"). The Task Force recommends that the professional community **not** use the term *fluency* to refer to *stuttering*. For example, it would be more precise to say or write: a diagnosis of "*stuttering*" rather than a diagnosis of "*fluency*," "client with *stuttering* " instead of "*fluency* client," and "*stuttering* treatment" instead of "*fluency* treatment." Those terms, however, may be appropriate in other contexts that do not include or relate to *stuttering* per se.

Fluency is used in the area of neurogenic communication disorders (i.e., aphasia) to refer to the perceived natural continuity and *rate* of spontaneous speech, even though there may be a substantial number of language errors (e.g., a "fluent aphasic" as opposed to a "nonfluent aphasic").

In the area of foreign language learning, *fluency* may refer to the general competence or facility with which a speaker can communicate orally in the new language(s) (e.g., "*fluent* in French"). In this usage, *fluency* is roughly equivalent to "overall spoken lan-

guage proficiency." In addition to this general usage, *fluency* also refers more specifically to the *rate*, continuity, *rhythm*, and *effort* with which the language is produced (e.g., "The speaker's knowledge of Russian vocabulary is adequate, but his *fluency* in spoken Russian is weak"). As noted by Wingate (1984), *fluency* typically refers to spoken language, but, presumably, it would be appropriate to refer to one's *fluency* in American Sign Language.

The Task Force proposes that the scientific community consider the value of the concepts of "motor *fluency*" (e.g., speech coordination variables related to *fluency* in a *stutterer*) versus "linguistic *fluency*" (e.g., lexical, syntactic, or semantic variables related to *fluency* in a foreign language speaker or a *clutterer*). Research is ongoing in these areas and may suggest other or better ways to account for the often conflicting, contradictory uses of the term *fluency*. In any case, appropriate descriptors or clarifiers should be used to minimize confusion regarding the use of the term.

3.2. Fluency Disorder. A fluency disorder is a "speech disorder" characterized by deviations in continuity, smoothness, rhythm, and/or effort with which phonologic, lexical, morphologic, and/or syntactic language units are spoken.

In recent years, the profession of speech-language pathology has adopted the term *fluency disorders* to denote a category of "speech disorders" (as opposed to "language disorders"), that includes such related disorders as *stuttering* and *cluttering* as well as the more specific categories of *neurogenic stuttering* and *psychogenic stuttering*. Indeed, the Special Interest Division responsible for these Guidelines deals with "*fluency* and *fluency disorders*." Specific disorders of *rate* (i.e., too fast, too slow, or too irregular) are generally considered to be *fluency disorders* as well, even though other disorders (e.g., word retrieval or insufficient vocabulary) might be present and even responsible for *rate* problems.

3.3. Disfluency. Disfluency refers to breaks in the continuity of producing phonologic, lexical, morphologic, and/or syntactic language units in oral speech.

The generic term *disfluency* refers to breaks that are normal, abnormal, or ambiguous (i.e., sometimes regarded as normal and sometimes abnormal). The most commonly regarded *normal disfluencies* are: hesitations or long pauses for language formulation (e.g., "This is our [*pause*] miscellaneous group"); word fillers (e.g., "The color is *like* red"), also known as "filled pauses"; nonword fillers (sometimes called interjections, e.g., "The color is *uh* red"); and phrase repetitions (e.g., "This is a—this is a problem"). The most common ambiguous *disfluencies* are whole word repetitions (e.g., "*I-I-I* want to go" or "This is a *better-better* solution"). The most commonly regarded abnormal *disfluencies* (i.e., *stutterings*) are: part-word (or sound/syllable) repetitions (e.g., "Look at the *buh-buh-ba*-baby"); prolongations (e.g., "*Sssssss*sometimes we stay home"); blockages (silent fixations/prolongations of articulatory postures) or <u>noticeable and unusually</u> long (tense/silent) pauses at unusual locations to postpone or avoid (e.g., "Give me a glass (*3-sec pause*) of water"); and any of the above categories when accompanied by decidedly greater than average duration, *effort*, tension, or struggle.

Although the term *disfluency* does not necessarily imply abnormality, it is often used synonymously with *stuttering* and, as noted in section 3.4, interchangeably with *dysfluency*. Clinicians often use *disfluency* to refer to *stuttering* for a number of reasons, including: (a) assuming it is perceived by clients to be, connotatively, a less negative term than *stuttering*, (b) believing it sounds more scientific or objective than *stuttering*, or (c) regarding it to be synonymous with *stuttering*. There is little empirical or logical support for any of these assumptions. Clinical researchers occasionally prefer the term *disfluency* to *stuttering* because they find it easier to make reliable judgments of all *disfluencies* than only those further judged to be *stutterings*.

"Normal developmental *disfluencies*" refer to higher than adult levels of *normal disfluencies* that occur in preschool children as they learn language normally. Approximately half of nonstuttering children go through an identifiable period of "increased normal developmental *disfluency*" during this time (Johnson & Associates, 1959).

Starkweather (1987) introduced the term *discontinuity* because it differentially refers to breaks in the continuity or flow of speech and not to other problems of *fluency*, such as a *rate* that is too slow. Given Starkweather's analysis, the Task Force concurs that the term *discontinuity* makes a useful distinction and, therefore, might result in more incisive use of terminology. Nevertheless, it chose to accord preference to the term *disfluency* (in spite of its misuses) because it is overwhelmingly the more popular term referring to breaks in continuity.

Nonfluency is sometimes used synonymously with *disfluency*.

3.4. Dysfluency. (Same as stuttering [see 3.5].)

According to Wingate (1984), the "dys" and "dis" prefixes are quite different. The "dys" prefix implies abnormality, such that a word beginning with "dys" denotes an abnormal condition. By contrast, the "dis" prefix denotes separation, negation, or signals a contrast with the morpheme that follows it. Wingate cites three of four dictionary references to support his view. It must be pointed out, however, that all dictionaries, such as the Oxford Unabridged Dictionary, do not show this distinction. Some hold that the "dys" prefix in the field of speech-language pathology implies an underlying, organic impairment whereas the "dis" prefix implies deviant behavior. Accepting the somewhat controversial assumption that the prefixes are different, *dysfluency* (or "abnormal *fluency*") is essentially synonymous with *stuttering*. However, most recent texts still prefer the term *stuttering*.

As noted, *dysfluency* is frequently used interchangeably with *disfluency* (see 3.3), although professional consensus suggests that the two terms are not necessarily synonymous.

3.5. Stuttering.

Given the diversity of professional opinion on what constitutes *stuttering*, the Task Force recommends that clinicians and researchers recognize and indicate which of the following four uses, or combinations thereof, of the term *stuttering* they refer to in their references to this *fluency disorder*. Two uses refer primarily to the <u>behavior</u> of *stuttering*, and two refer primarily to <u>individuals</u> who manifest the behavior. The first two are essentially perceptual definitions (i.e., defined by a listener), the first from a specific symptom orientation and the second from a nonspecific orientation. The third defines *stuttering* in terms of private experience of the person who *stutters*, and the fourth focuses on the suspected cause or nature of *stuttering*. In all cases, *stuttering* refers to a communication disorder related to speech *fluency* that generally begins during childhood (but, occasionally, as late as early adulthood). Some individuals refer to this typical *stuttering* as "developmental stuttering." Others refer to *stuttering* as a "syndrome," focusing thereby on a set of symptoms that may coexist in any *stuttering* individual. *Neurogenic stuttering* and *psychogenic stuttering* are special cases that are not subtypes of typical or "developmental"*stuttering*, despite the widespread use of these terms (see 3.12 and 3.13).

3.5.1. Stuttering refers to speech events that contain monosyllabic whole-word repetitions, part-word repetitions, audible sound prolongations, or silent fixations or blockages. These may or may not

be accompanied by accessory (secondary) behaviors (i.e., behaviors used to escape and/or avoid these speech events).

This definition implies that certain categories of symptoms or *disfluencies* (see below) can generally be classified as abnormal and that others can be considered normal. With this definition, the fact that specific examples within any of the above *disfluency* categories may be variously perceived as normal or abnormal is generally disregarded. Also, the category of monosyllabic whole word repetitions is not always considered *stuttering*, depending on such variables as age of the client, locus within the utterance, duration, and other factors. This definition implies that *stuttering* occurs on specific language units (e.g., words or syllables).

This definition is intuitively appealing to clinicians for it renders *stuttering* a quantifiable phenomenon, suggests specific targets of treatment (i.e., the *disfluency* categories with the most *stuttering*), and allows for careful clinical descriptions of *accessory (secondary) behaviors* (see 3.6). It also has appeal for research, especially in determining beforehand which subjects will and will not be included in *stuttering* groups.

3.5.2. Stuttering consists of speech events that are reliably perceived to be stuttering by observers.

This definition relies on operationalism, that is, defining a difficult concept by the operations used to measure it. Specifically, the definition implies that a listener or conversation partner does not require a specific orientation to identify instances of *stuttering*. One does so because he or she knows the language in question and can therefore identify abnormalities in its production. The operations involved are those that are quantifiable and that specify reliability assessments. The definer must demonstrate a reasonable degree of agreement with other "judges" on the measures taken, as well as with himself or herself in repeated assessments, in identifying specific instances of *stuttering*. This definition grants credibility to the obvious situation that one does not need to be trained to recognize a *stuttering* problem. No doubt, speech events regarded as *stuttering* in the previous definition are responsible for most judgments of *stuttering*. Nevertheless, with this symptom-nonspecific definition, a "moment of *stuttering*" may, in some circumstances, be attributed to *disfluency* categories that, in other circumstances, would be regarded as normal, and vice versa. As in the previous definition, *stutter-*

ing is quantifiable and allows for careful descriptions of *accessory (secondary) behaviors*.

This operational definition has appeal for clinicians who choose to use an approach in treatment requiring "on line" counts or immediate consequences or feedback to be provided immediately after each "moment of *stuttering*." It is also particularly appealing to researchers who require reliable measures of *stuttering*.

3.5.3. Stuttering refers to the private, personal experience of an involuntary loss of control by the person who stutters. As such, it often affects the effectiveness of the speaker's communication.

This definition focuses on the experience of the person who stutters rather than judgments of clinicians, observers, or theoreticians. The most vocal advocate of this view is Perkins (1990), who wrote that "stuttering is the involuntary disruption of a continuing attempt to produce a spoken utterance" in which "involuntary" is understood to reflect the speaker's feeling of "loss of control." This orientation allows the clinician to appreciate the difference between "real" and "faked" *stuttering* and have a more inclusive definition for the client who claims to be a "*stutterer*" but overtly "*stutters*" only on rare occasions.

This definition has particular appeal to persons, especially adults, with a history of *stuttering* themselves because it describes what they experience as a *stuttering*. It has been regarded by many to have questionable use alone in clinical and research efforts because objective, replicable judgments of *stuttering* are difficult or impossible to obtain.

3.5.4. Stuttering refers to disordered speech that occurs as the result of: (a) certain physiological, neurological, or psychological deviations; (b) certain linguistic, affective, behavioral, or cognitive processes; or (c) some combination thereof.

This is not a definition per se. Instead, it refers to numerous definitions such as the following: "Stuttering is an anticipatory, apprehensive, hypertonic avoidance reaction" (Johnson, Brown, Curtis, Edney, & Keaster, 1967); "Stuttering occurs when the forward flow of speech is interrupted by a motorically disrupted sound, syllable, or word or by the speaker's reactions thereto" (Van Riper, 1982); or ". . .stuttering constitutes a covert repair reaction to some flaw in the speech plan" (Kolk & Postma, 1997).

These definitions focus on theory construction and address the questions, "What causes *stuttering*?" and/or "What is the nature of *stuttering*?" Such definitions, to the extent that they balance available knowledge with available research technology, can lead to testable hypotheses about the nature of *stuttering*.

Cause-based definitions are appealing to many *stuttering* clients, especially those seeking "answers" or insights into their disorder. In some cases such definitions suggest new or specific approaches to treatment. By contrast, they are generally not suitable for measuring *stuttering* behaviors in clinical or research settings.

3.5.5. Other Comments

As with the case of the "general" definition provided, a number of definitions of *stuttering* include elements of more than one of the above variants. For example, the World Health Organization (1977) defines *stuttering* as "disorders of rhythm of speech in which the individual knows precisely what he wishes to say, but at the time is unable to say it because of involuntary, repetitive prolongation or cessation of a sound." The *Diagnostic and Statistical Manual of Mental Disorders* (4th ed., rev., 1994; DSM-IV) indicates that "the essential feature of stuttering is a disturbance in the normal fluency and time patterning of speech that is inappropriate for the individual's age." Stuttering is characterized by "frequent repetitions or prolongations of sounds or syllables," but also can include "interjections … broken words (e.g., pauses within a word) … audible or silent blocking (filled or unfilled pauses in speech) … circumlocutions (e.g., word substitutions to avoid problematic words) … and monosyllable whole word repetitions (e.g., 'I-I-I-I see him')." In addition, the DSM-IV requires that "the disturbance in fluency interferes with academic or occupational achievement or with social communication" and all these difficulties exceed those usually associated with a "speech-motor or sensory deficit," if present.

Many individuals who *stutter* acquire maladaptive patterns of thinking and feeling, sufficiently common to be identified as frequent covert aspects of *stuttering*. For example, a child who *stutters* may adopt the belief that speaking is inherently difficult (Bloodstein, 1995). Those who *stutter* for a number of years often acquire the negative self-concept of "*stutterer*," leading them to adopt other beliefs and attitudes consistent with this self-concept (Cooper, 1990; Peters & Guitar, 1991). Also, many *stuttering* children and adults report fear or anxiety about speaking, or the prospect of speaking; frustration from the excessive time and effort imposed by *stuttered* speech; embarrassment, shame, or guilt following *stuttering*

episodes; and even hostility toward other conversation partners (Van Riper, 1982).

Stuttering is often used in lay usage to refer to *disfluencies* (see 3.3), both normal and abnormal. Also, many nonstutterers report that they have experienced *stuttering* of a sort they would regard as abnormal a few times in their lives.

In 1993, as the result of the influence of a number of consumer and self-help groups, the American Speech-Language-Hearing Association (ASHA) adopted a policy in which person-first language is to be used in lieu of direct labels (Executive Board Meeting Minutes, 1993). According to the policy, *stutterer* is regarded as potentially insensitive to the individual who manifests the problem of *stuttering*. Therefore, authors are required to use the term *person who stutters* instead of *stutterer*. Recent articles have tended to use abbreviations (e.g., PWS for *person who stutters* or CWS for *child who stutters)* to avoid the awkwardness inherent in using the longer versions.

No systematic research was carried out to support the ASHA "person-first" policy. Since its inception, limited research has shown that person-first labeling may or may not be perceived less negatively by individuals with speech-language-hearing impairments, parents of such clients, speech-language pathology students, and the public. In the case of the terms *stutterer*, *stammerer*, or *clutterer*, the results do not clearly indicate that these direct labels consistently communicate greater sensitivity than the person-first versions (Robinson & Robinson, 1996; St. Louis, 1998). More research is needed, but the available findings cast doubt on both the need and wisdom underlying the recent changes in terminology. Person-first labeling warrants serious consideration when referring to specific individuals, especially in clinical situations, for it implies that there is much more to a person than the fact that he or she *stutters*. On the other hand, given the fact that many nonstutterers report that they have occasionally "*stuttered*," the *person who stutters* nomenclature may create ambiguity in descriptions of subjects in research reports wherein the traditional distinction between *stutterer* and *nonstutterer* is important. Until additional research is completed, clinicians or researchers will—and possibly should—use their own discretion in the use of those terms.

Stammering is synonymous with *stuttering* and is the common term for the disorder in Great Britain. In North America, the term *stammering* is rarely used by speech-language pathologists.

3.6. Accessory (Secondary) Behaviors. Accessory (or secondary) behaviors include the entire range of reactions, strategies, "tricks," and avoidance or escape behaviors that stutterers perform either when they stutter or in anticipation or fear of stuttering.

Accessory (secondary) behaviors are typically considered to be reactions to *stuttering* that are reinforced by their initial consequences, which, according to the user, reduce the *stuttering* abnormality (escape) or prevent or delay its occurrence (avoidance/postponement). *Accessory (secondary) behaviors* are considered to be learned (although there is some evidence that some may not be learned), and the *stutterer* may or may not be aware of their presence. They include such categories as: "avoidance behaviors" (e.g., not speaking when one wants to [as in class discussions] or substituting synonyms for feared words or circumlocuting/paraphrasing the intended utterance), "postponement devices" (e.g., stalling by using nonword or word fillers or simply waiting to attempt to talk), "timing devices" or "starters" (e.g., blinking the eyes, taking a short gasp, or getting a "running start" in order to begin to say a feared word), "disguise reactions" (e.g., covering one's mouth or faking a cough in order to hide the fact that one is stuttering), "interrupter devices" (e.g., jerking the head or grimacing to release from a long block), and "searching movements" (e.g., using the schwa or inappropriate vowel or altering the rate of repeated sounds or syllables). In some cases, evidence of "struggle" (see 3.8) may be regarded as an *accessory (secondary) behavior*.

In general, the word "accessory" (or "secondary") implies that the above listed behaviors and strategies accompany the core features of *stuttering* and that a causal account for these behaviors (i.e., learning) is implied. By contrast, when *stuttering* is considered to be a clinical syndrome, its affective, behavioral, and cognitive aspects (including strategies to hide and avoid the occurrence of *stuttering*) are considered to be integral components of the disorder rather than "accessory" (or "secondary") behaviors.

Accessory (secondary) behaviors are also known as "secondary mannerisms," "secondaries," "concomitant behaviors," or "extraneous behaviors."

3.7. Rate. Rate refers to the speed with which sounds, syllables, or words are spoken.

Speech *rate* is typically expressed in words or syllables per minute. Generally, only the periods of time in which the speaker is actually talking are included in calculating *rate*, and these include normal pauses. (Most of these normal pauses are less than

1 second; longer inter-utterance pauses [e.g., 2 seconds or more] are typically excluded from rate assessments. There are reasonable exceptions to excluding long pauses in rate assessments, e.g., when the evaluator wishes to consider the time taken up by long pauses that are associated with avoidance. In such cases, the time spent actually stuttering is occasionally reported as well.) Some researchers use the measure of "articulation *rate*" (also known as "phone *rate*" or "phoneme *rate*"), which is calculated from short periods of fluent speech that are free of perceptible pauses. This measure is often reported in syllables per second.

3.8. Effort. Effort refers to the amount of perceived exertion a speaker experiences during speaking.

Every speech act requires the speaker to exert some *effort*. The degree of *effort* required varies with such aspects as the speaker's familiarity with the language, topic, and listener(s); interference from internal and external sources; and individual differences in the capacity for fluent speech. The speaker's total *effort* includes both physiological and psychological components. Moreover, physiological and psychological *effort* interact with each other as in the cases wherein heightened emotion or certain thoughts result in excessive muscle tension. Similarly, cautious or overcontrolled speech may be characterized by inappropriate and/or excessive tension levels. "Struggle" is a special case of *effort* and refers to speech events that are characterized by unusual and/or excessive amounts of (physiological and/or psychological) *effort* during the production of some—but generally not all—sounds, words, or longer utterances. Effort can be considered both from the perspective of the speaker (i.e., the level of effort experienced during speech) or from the perspective of the listener (i.e., the degree of effort the listener attributes to the speaker's performance). It should be noted that some authorities prefer the term "ease" to *effort* because *fluency* generally has a connotation of "easy" rather than "hard" or "effortful."

3.9. Suprasegmental Features. Suprasegmental features are dimensions of speech that extend across phoneme or allophone (i.e., "segment") boundaries, and include such things as rhythm, prosody, melody, and inflection.

Certain prosodic features, such as intonation patterns that extend across several segments, are suprasegmental in nature. Similarly, an alteration of stress on a compound word (e.g., base'ball versus baseball') is a suprasegmental feature change.

3.9.1. *Rhythm.* **Rhythm refers to the pattern (timing and duration) of stressed and unstressed syllables in speech.**

Although related to "continuity" and *rate*, *rhythm* is more specific. It refers to the degree that a speaker's pattern of syllable stress in words and sentences is similar to a standard or predicted pattern. In other words, normal *rhythm* refers to maintaining a perceptibly appropriate pattern of "beats" and pauses at an acceptable *rate*. Deviations in *rhythm* may be perceived as variations in the "regularity of *rate*." Different languages have different characteristic *rhythms*, sometimes readily recognized by individuals listening to a conversation in a language they do not know. Moreover, the same language may have several normal variations in *rhythm*. For example, it is possible for a speaker to produce speech characterized by normal continuity and *rate*, but which violates the conversational stress pattern of the language or specific dialect in question (e.g., General American English). One such case pertains to numerous English speakers from India and Pakistan, who are often perceived to be quite fluent but not easily understood by native English speakers from North America unfamiliar with their variant of English. In this case, differences in the *rhythm* of the variants of English are partly responsible for the difficulty in understanding.

3.9.2. *Prosody.* **Prosody refers collectively to syllable stress, juncture, and intonation contours in speech.**

Prosody is related to *rhythm* in that both concepts include consideration of patterns of syllable stress and pauses. *Prosody* also includes the element of fundamental frequency changes related to intonation. Syllable stress refers to greater intensity, slightly higher fundamental frequency, and longer durations on certain syllables, as in "I' live in the white house" versus "I *live*' in the white house." Juncture, among other things, refers to subtle differences in the length of pauses between words, as in "I live in the *white house.*" versus "I live in the *White House*" (dwelling of the U.S. president). Intonation contours refer to meaningful frequency variations on words, phrases, and longer utterances, as in "I *live¬* in the white house" (i.e., "I do live there") versus "I *live* (in the white house ?" (i.e., Do I live there?"). As a term for description of some aspect of *fluency*, *prosody* suffers from a lack of agreed-on specificity.

3.10. *Naturalness.* **Naturalness refers to the degree to which speech (and language) sounds like that of normal, native speakers.**

Naturalness is a global measure and has been typically determined by playing samples of speech to a group of normal listeners and asking them to judge how *natural* the speech sounds according to a 9-point equal-appearing interval scale (Martin, Haroldson, & Triden, 1984). In ways that are not well understood, *naturalness* as a measure in *fluency disorders* is related to ratings of overall disorder severity, *fluency*, *rhythm*, *rate*, and *prosody*. Whereas persons with mild *stuttering* may have "natural-sounding speech," the degree of *naturalness* perceived by the listener usually decreases (i.e., becomes more "unnatural") as *stuttering* becomes more severe.

3.11. *Cluttering.* **Cluttering is a fluency disorder characterized by a rapid and/or irregular speech rate, excessive disfluencies, and often other symptoms such as language or phonological errors and attention deficits.**

Cluttering is a term that describes a constellation of symptoms, including *fluency* problems. Most of the early writing on *cluttering* grew out of the European traditions of phoniatrics and logopedics. Except for isolated publications, *cluttering* was generally ignored in North America until recently. The definition of *cluttering* is not clearly established, but most current authorities agree that deficits in *fluency*, *rate*, and coexisting disorders of language and/or articulation are nearly always present. Problems in such areas as attention, activity level, reading, and handwriting suggest strong parallels between *cluttering* and "learning disabilities" and "attention-deficit/hyperactivity disorders."

Generally, the *disfluencies* observed in clutterers consist of those typically regarded as "normal" or "ambiguous," referred to earlier. *Cluttering* may occur alone as a *fluency disorder*, but it more frequently coexists with *stuttering*.

3.12. *Neurogenic Stuttering.* **Neurogenic stuttering refers to stuttering, often transient, that began with—or is maintained as a result of—a specific, identifiable neurological insult or lesion.**

Generally, *neurogenic stuttering* is observed in adults who have undergone confirmed brain damage. An infrequently occurring disorder, it has been observed in individuals who have lesions in diverse areas of the central nervous system (e.g., Helm-Estabrooks, 1993). *Neurogenic stuttering* has been labeled variously as "acquired stuttering," "stuttering secondary to brain damage," and "cortical stuttering." Some in the professional community question whether *neurogenic stuttering* is a valid diagnostic entity.

3.13. *Psychogenic Stuttering.* Psychogenic stuttering is stuttering that is clearly related to psychopathology.

Psychogenic stuttering refers to *stuttering* that is the primary symptom of some form of verifiable psychopathology, such as a neurotic conversion disorder (e.g., Roth, Aronson, & Davis, 1989). Excluded from this somewhat questionable category is *stuttering* that began after a psychologically traumatic event because, in most cases, the *stuttering* symptoms continue to develop in much the same way as do symptoms of *stuttering* that began in childhood after no such traumatic event. The Task Force cautions researchers and clinicians to use the term *psychogenic stuttering* only in cases in which it is clearly related to diagnosed psychopathology. Some in the professional community question the validity of *psychogenic stuttering* as a diagnostic entity.

4. References

American Psychiatric Association. (1994). *Diagnostic and statistical manual of mental disorders* (4th ed.). Washington, DC: Author.

Bloodstein, O. (1995). *A handbook on stuttering* (5th ed.). San Diego, CA: Singular.

Cooper, E. B. (1990). *Understanding stuttering: Information for parents.* Chicago: National Easter Seal Society.

Executive Board Meeting Minutes (1993, December). *Asha,* 35, 128.

Helm-Estabrooks, N. (1993). Stuttering associated with acquired neurological disorders. In R. F. Curlee (Ed.), *Stuttering and related disorders of fluency* (pp. 205–219). New York: Thieme Medical Publishers.

Johnson, W., & Associates (1959). *The onset of stuttering: Research findings and implications.* Minneapolis: University of Minnesota Press.

Johnson, W., Brown, S. F., Curtis, J. F., Edney, C. W., & Keaster, J. (1967). *Speech handicapped school children* (3rd ed.). New York: Harper & Row.

Kolk, H., & Postma, A. (1997). Stuttering as a covert repair phenomenon. In R. F. Curlee & G. M. Siegel (Eds.), *Nature and treatment of stuttering: New directions* (2nd ed., pp. 182–203). Boston: Allyn & Bacon.

Martin, R. R., Haroldson, S. K., & Triden, K. A. (1984). Stuttering and speech naturalness. *Journal of Speech and Hearing Disorders, 49,* 53–58.

Perkins, W. H. (1990). What is stuttering? *Journal of Speech and Hearing Disorders, 55,* 370–382.

Peters, T. J., & Guitar, B. (1991). *Stuttering: An integrated approach to its nature and treatment.* Baltimore: Williams & Wilkins.

Robinson, B., & Robinson, B. (1996). *Person-first language and attitudes toward individuals who stutter.* Paper presented at the annual Convention of the American Speech-Language-Hearing Association, Seattle, WA.

Roth, C. R., Aronson, A. E., & Davis, L. J. (1989). Clinical studies in psychogenic stuttering of adult onset. *Journal of Speech and Hearing Disorders, 54,* 634–646.

Starkweather, C. W. (1987). *Fluency and stuttering.* Englewood Cliffs, NJ: Prentice-Hall.

St. Louis, K. O. (1998). Person-first labeling and stuttering. *Journal of Fluency Disorders, 23,* 1–24.

Van Riper, C. (1982). *The nature of stuttering* (2nd ed.). Englewood Cliffs, NJ: Prentice-Hall.

Wingate, M. E. (1984). Fluency, disfluency, dysfluency, and stuttering. *Journal of Fluency Disorders, 17,* 163–168.

World Health Organization. (1977). *Manual of the international statistical classification of diseases, injuries, and causes of death* (Vol. 1). Geneva: World Health Organization.

Why tell your story?

"Taking Stock" implies stopping to look and think carefully about what is happening in our lives, where we are going, and what we have or need. There is generally an underlying question, "Are things going well?" "Do we need to make some change?" Ordinarily we are forced to take stock when a tragedy strikes such as the loss of a loved one, an unplanned or sudden move, a natural disaster, and so on. But periodic taking stock can be an important part of staying in touch with ourselves day-to-day, week-to-week, month-to-month, year-to-year, or even "chapter-to-chapter" in our lives. It is no accident that each New Year is often associated with resolutions to change or to do better. And, isn't making serious New Year's resolutions always preceded by taking stock?

I submit that it is useful and therapeutic to take stock of our stuttering from time to time as well. As noted in *Chapter 1: Introduction,* White and Epston talk not about "people having problems" but about "problems having people." This means that "stuttering" (or being a "stutterer" or "person who stutters") carries with it all kinds of societal or cultural expectations and assumptions that relate to anyone with that problem or label. And these attitudes are applied 1) whether or not they fit your situation and 2) whether or not they are even true. Chances are that you hold many of the same expectations and assumptions that the people around you do, whether you know it or not.

I recommend that you tell your story, especially if you have never confronted your stuttering in therapy, but even if you have had successful therapy or believe that you have overcome your stuttering. Why? When you tell your own story you just might discover which of those expectations and assumptions underlie or guide your own beliefs and actions. Sometimes you need to hear or read your story—the one you told—before some of those insights come to you. Your story, of course, changes throughout your life, so the story you tell now is not the same as the one you might have told a decade ago or would tell a decade hence. When you tell your story—for the first or the fifth time—you are taking stock.

Having told your story, if you chose to do so, you could begin to change some of your own expectations and assumptions. One way would be to utilize some of the principles of "narrative therapy." In this framework, it becomes possible to change your story by exploring alternate explanations and adopting new conceptual paradigms. For example, in telling your story, suppose you discovered that you are fairly comfortable with your stuttering, but you see a pattern of not seeking promotions in your job, promotions for which you would probably compete very well. Suppose as well that you learned from your story that speaking to new customers has always required more effort than interacting with old customers or co-workers, even though you always could interact with new customers if you had to. You suspect it is related to an old gut-level feeling that your stuttering makes you not quite as good as you would otherwise be. Furthermore, you listened to your story and concluded that you have assumed for a long time that you should not be placed in a position in your company where your stuttering might negatively affect its profitability or growth potential. As a loyal employee, naturally you would not have sought promotions that would place you in the position in which, by virtue of your stuttering, you might possibly lose some new accounts or not articulate your decisions to others about future directions the company should take.

If all of the above were true, it is indeed possible that you might discover that, given your abilities, knowledge, and experience, there is no reason to accept the assumption that stuttering reflects in any negative way on your potential in a leadership role. And, if this scenario were true, it would follow that your "story of stuttering," after changing your assumptions and expectations for yourself, would become quite different.

How can you tell your story?

Probably the easiest way to tell your story is to sit down and relate it to another person who is genuinely interested in you. That person could be a wife or husband, a sister or brother, a child or parent, or a close friend. It could also be a speech-language pathologist, counselor, or religious leader. Whoever the person might be, you will basically arrange for him or her to interview you. Unless this taking stock exercise is part of an evaluation or treatment component of speech therapy or counseling, you will probably need to "make an appointment" with your "interviewer." I recommend that you arrange a quiet place alone for the two of you and also arrange that you will not be interrupted for about an hour. This all may seem terribly awkward, but most close family members or friends would be honored that you trusted them enough to listen and ask questions about your experiences with stuttering.

Let me provide an example. For the past five years, I have asked my students to interview someone who has personal experience with stuttering. I have also asked them to check with their families and friends if they don't personally know someone to ask. Amazingly, about ten students have ended up interviewing someone in their immediate family (usually a parent) who they never knew had stuttered. And in most cases, the interview became a watershed event in their relationship, drawing the student and family member much closer than before.

Another good way to tell your story, if you are comfortable doing so, is to tell it to a supportive group. No doubt many stutterers would not find this comfortable, but some of you who are not particularly sensitive about a current or past stuttering problem—or others of you who are sick and tired of keeping your problem locked up inside—might actually find it easier than talking to one person. The setting might be a stuttering self-help or support group or a number of close friends who get together regularly. Be sure to pick a group that has a history of supporting one another and one that can talk about things beyond the usual "safe" topics of conversation. Another possibility is to tell your story in a "speech" for a class or "Toastmasters" club. Most of us who have done this have been amazed and heartened by the wonderful response we get. I was once richly blessed to have been part of a panel of eight "recovered stutterers" who told our stories to about 600 speech-language pathologists at our national convention. In over 25 years of attending conventions, I have never participated in or attended a session in which there was so much energy, excitement, optimism, and power.

> "I had no idea that he felt the way he did about his stuttering. He has talked about it with me on occasion but never in this depth. The interview gave me a better understanding of what he goes through and has gone through personally." —*graduate student in speech-language pathology who interviewed her husband*

Finally, it is even possible to tell your story to yourself. For some people, turning their thoughts and feelings into words helps them to clarify, define, and put things into better perspective. This may feel very strange at first, but if you really want to tell your story, sometimes it is the surest way to do so. One further advantage of this approach is that if you stutter a lot with other people, you will almost certainly be able to tell your story to yourself with little or no stuttering. If you tape record yourself, you also may find it interesting to hear how fluent you might become. Finally, you might be thinking about seeking speech therapy for yourself. After deciding upon a speech-language pathologist, it could be very helpful to be able to give this person your tape to listen to before or during the evaluation process.

Of course, as I noted, a speech-language pathologist might suggest you tell your story as part of an evaluation or therapy. This would probably occur in the clinician's office or therapy setting, but it could well be a pre-evaluation exercise that you could complete on your own and then share it with the speech-language pathologist, especially if you needed to travel a considerable distance to the evaluation.

Importantly, in any of these situations I strongly suggest you have a tape recorder turned on to record what you are saying. Telling *and hearing* your story can be useful. If you choose to record it—and I hope you do—there are a few critically important procedures to follow. For many people, these suggestions may seem annoyingly obvious, but I have seen too many interviews become lost forever because insufficient attention was paid to one or more of the following common sense principles.

Pick a quiet place for recording or, if the environment is not quiet, use a good lapel microphone that can be directed to your voice.

Make sure the tape recorder works in advance by recording and playing back a short segment.

Make sure the tape recorder has new batteries in it or—even better—is one that can be plugged in. If batteries are to be used, it is wise to have a spare set of new ones.

Buy one or two *new* tapes of good quality to use. ("Voice" tapes are a little better than "music" tapes if you have a choice.)

Make sure the "record" button is pushed—not just the "play" button—after you test the tape recorder.

Use the "pause" button if you need to stop the tape during the interview rather than the "stop" button to avoid the problem suggested above.

Arrange to have the built-in or remote microphone of the tape recorder close to you—not several feet away. Don't worry if it does not pick up the voice(s) of the other person/people well.

Do not touch the microphone or the microphone cord anytime the tape recorder is on. It will make noise that can completely drown out your speech.

Turn the tape over or put in a new one when one side is finished. Check from time to time to see if you need to do so.

Make a copy of the tape in case one gets lost. This is especially important if you plan to loan or send it to someone else, even your speech-language pathologist.

There is no prescription of how long your story should be. Most people are able to tell their stories of stuttering in a half-hour to an hour. Yours might be shorter (e.g., if you are giving a speech or telling a group) or longer than that (e.g., if you want to get all the parts of it said by yourself). If you don't finish in your planned time, you can always resume at a later time, even if you have to do it alone.

Once finished, what should you do with your tape? If you are a "private person," you might feel most comfortable telling and listening to your story a few times and then disposing of the tape. But it has been my experience that your story will contain very important, uniquely personal, and potentially irreplaceable aspects of your history, all of which are worth keeping. Even if you don't want anyone to know about your story now, as that story evolves and changes, you may find that you choose to share it with others to help educate the public, to help others who stutter, or to pass on part of your own legacy. You also may want to tell your story again some time in the future and then go back and learn what has changed since this telling.

Some people don't feel comfortable telling their stories out loud. If this statement describes you, you can write your story down. Writing your story should not be viewed as writing a theme or a literary short story. It should be viewed as a way to simply record your thoughts, no matter if they make any sense to you or someone else later. You should write just as you might talk. Write what comes to mind, not worrying about spelling, grammar, punctuation, paragraphs, wording, and so on. Again, if you choose this option, I suggest you select times to write that are quiet and free from serious interruptions, although breaks will not be as distracting as if you were telling your story aloud. If you write easier than you type, use a pencil or pen. If not, type the story. (Just be sure to save it often if you are using a computer!)

As with a tape, you may not want anyone to read what you wrote. If you feel strongly about this, you will protect what you wrote and not share it. But, again, I would argue that you should not destroy it. Seal a printed copy of your story in an envelope, and keep it in a safe place. And, as noted earlier, you may find that you wish to use your story for later taking stock activities, therapy, educating the public, helping others, or in your own personal history or memoir. Make a photocopy as a backup.

There are numerous additional resources to help you if you choose to write your story of stuttering, or even your life story. Examples include Ira Progoff's *Intensive Journal® process; Personal Journaling* (a magazine); and dozens of how-to books identified by such key words as personal history, memoir, and life story. Populore Publishing Company, publisher of this book, is a company dedicated to helping ordinary people preserve their stories. Its *Put It In Writing: Guide for Populore Narratives* can help you write short narratives about different parts and memories of your life (for information: http://www.populore.com).

Ready? Get started!

At this point, if you can tell your story without further help, do it! There is no need to read any further until you have finished. Spontaneous stories straight from your mouth or your pen are almost always the most personal, the most revealing, and the most valuable.

If you are puzzled about where to start, read on.

Getting started in an oral interview or written narrative can be a serious hurdle. Do you start your story with your first memory of stuttering? Do you begin with the first thing that comes to your mind? There are no rules whatever in this matter, but I would suggest that you avoid trying to do a neat chronology, starting from your earliest memory of stuttering and progressing to the present. Of course, chronology is usually present in stories, but if you try to get it all, you will find that it could take months or years to tell your story.

Instead, I suggest thinking about any or all of the "partial lead sentence" statements in the *Telling Your Story Worksheet*, a copy of which is provided. Try to simply talk or write about any of your own experiences these partial sentences bring to mind. Start anywhere in the list with a statement that seems easy to talk about. There is definitely no recommended order. If you find yourself going off on a tangent, stay with it; it means you are becoming spontaneous. When you can't think of anything else on one topic, move to another. The rationale for this exercise is very simple. If you are talking or writing with interest or passion about a stuttering-related experience or insight that a statement made you think of, it is probably important. Chances are, you would not have much to say about something that was not important to you.

Remember, it's your story. If you are telling it to someone else—or a group—and they have a lot of questions, don't allow yourself to get sidetracked if you don't want to. On the other hand, be open to their questions; they may lead you in an interesting, fruitful direction.

Start your story now if you want.

No doubt, you are already thinking of some of the topics you would like to cover when you tell you story. Following is a *Telling Your Story Worksheet*. It contains context information for later reference and some partial lead sentences. There are also three blank pages for you to jot down some ideas or to even begin writing your story. As you begin your journey of telling your story, you may want to obtain a special notebook—or a box to store loose notebook paper—where you can do your original writing or where you can make notes from tape recordings.

Telling Your Story Worksheet

A **Taking Stock** Self-Study Exercise • Kenneth O. St. Louis, Ph.D.

Name: _____ Age: _____ Date: _____

Setting: _____

How did you tell your story?

_____ To another person orally. Who? _____

_____ To a group orally. Describe? _____

_____ To myself orally.

_____ To my speech-language pathologist orally. Who? _____

_____ To myself in writing.

_____ To my speech-language pathologist in writing. Who? _____

If told orally, is your story on tape?

_____ Yes. Type of tape? _____

_____ No.

How do you think your story can help you?

_____ Listen to or read the story myself for deeper insights.

_____ Share my story with someone else. Who? _____

_____ Give a copy to my speech-language pathologist.

_____ Share my story with a self-help or support group.

_____ Use to compare my progress at some later date.

_____ Keep it in my personal mementos.

_____ Other. What? _____

Suggested lead sentences to help you get started or to tell more of your story.

My stuttering is…

I remember stuttering being especially bad when…

In school, my stuttering…

At work, I have found that stuttering…

In my family, stuttering was…

Of all the things I have been told about my stuttering, I most remember…

If you stutter, you know that…

If you don't stutter, you probably don't understand that…

Talking to strangers is…

As a child, my speech was…

Because I stutter(ed), I really care(d) about…

If I had it to do over, when I stutter(ed), I would…

Another stutterer I met or knew…

The worst thing about stuttering is…

The best thing about stuttering is…

One thing about stuttering that always upsets me is…

My clearest memory of stuttering is…

If you are talking to someone who stutterers, don't…

When I was alone, I often thought that stuttering…

When other people were having fun, because I stuttered, I usually…

When I was a child, the other kids thought my stuttering was…

What I think caused my stuttering was…

Since I stutter(ed), using the telephone is (was)…

When most people think about stuttering, they…

Speech therapy for me is (was)…

Of all the things you could have happen to you, stuttering…

My story…

My story...

My story…

Additional Resources

If you would like assistance in how to preserve your story, either in its present form, in a rewritten and professionally laid out form like the stories in *Living with Stuttering: Stories, Basics, Resources, and Hope,* or in some other form (e.g., in a special portfolio or transcribed from a tape recording), please contact Populore Publishing Company, PO Box 4382, Morgantown, WV 26504.

Please note that individual copies—as well as quantity packets—of Populore's Taking Stock materials in *Appendices G and H* are available. This includes the *Telling Your Story Worksheet, SL♦ILP-S, SL♦ILP-S/R, SL♦ILP-S Scoring Summary Sheet,* instructions for using all of these forms, and related discussion. For information, request a Triumph Series catalogue or see p. 255.

Taking and scoring the
St. Louis Inventory of Life Perspectives and Stuttering (SL•ILP-S).

The best way to begin "taking stock" of your stuttering is to tell your story (see *Appendix G: Taking Stock: Telling Your Story of Stuttering*). As part of—or instead of—that exercise, you might wish to fill out a questionnaire that can quickly tell you something about how much your stuttering affects your life and a few things about how you view your past or present speech problem. I developed the *St. Louis Inventory of Life Perspectives and Stuttering (SL•ILP-S)*, a self-study inventory for people who stutter, to provide this kind of information. It has thirteen questions designed to assess three areas: your stuttering and its effects on you; your interest in others who stutter; and your health and life satisfaction. You can score each item on a scale from one to nine, or choose "I don't know." In addition, I created the *St. Louis Inventory of Life Perspectives and Stuttering/Recollections (SL•ILP-S/R)* which asks the same questions, but for a time in the past.

There are no right or wrong answers on the inventories. Each is simply a way to take a quick look at what bothers you about your stuttering, and how important stuttering is in your life compared to other concerns. They give you benchmarks to compare your ongoing progress in dealing with your stuttering.

I recommend that you first take the *SL•ILP-S* for the current time. Then, if you are an adult, take the *SL•ILP-S/R* twice more, doing your best to remember how you would have filled it out when you were about ten years old and then also when you were in high school.

After you have filled out each version, transfer your ratings to the *SL•ILP-S Scoring Summary Sheet*. Start with the *second* line (for question number 1) on the *Scoring Summary Sheet* and go through the inventory and circle the numbers on the *Scoring Summary Sheet* that you circled on your inventory. (Use squares and triangles for your responses on the *SL•ILP-S/R.*) Enter the *13th* item at the *top* on the first line.

Once you have transferred all your scores to the *Scoring Summary Sheet*, connect the circles in each row with lines to make a graph of your results. If you also filled out the *SL♦ILP-S/R*, use a different color to connect the squares and another to connect the triangles, or different styles of lines, such as dots or dashes. Next, total the scores for items 1, 2, 3, 4, 5, 6, and 13 to determine Total Effect Scores. (Item 7 is omitted from this score because it is possible that you may not be aware of the effects of your stuttering on those around you.)

In general, scores on the left side of the *SL♦ILP-S Scoring Summary Sheet*, graphs that move toward the left, and lower Total Effect Scores indicate an individual who is more accepting of—and more comfortable with—stuttering than those with scores or graphs on the right side of the *Summary Sheet* and higher Total Effect Scores. Although this is a self-study inventory, you may wish to compare your Total Effect Scores to those of other stutterers who have filled out the *SL♦ILP-S*. Some summary data is provided at the end of this appendix.

Please note that individual copies—as well as quantity packets—of the Taking Stock materials in this and the previous appendix are available. This includes the *SL♦ILP-S, SL♦ILP-S/R, SL♦ILP-S Scoring Summary Sheet, Telling Your Story Worksheet*, instructions for using all of these forms, and related discussion. For information, request a Triumph Series catalogue from Populore Publishing Company, PO Box 4382, Morgantown, West Virginia 26504.

Sample forms and a hypothetical example.

Following are two sample copies of the *St. Louis Inventory of Life Perspectives and Stuttering*, the first one referring to the present time (*SL♦ILP-S*) and the second one referring to recollections of some time in the past (*SL♦ILP-S/R*). Both have been filled out by a hypothetical person who stutters, Jerome, once at his current age of thirty-two and once when he was about ten years old.

Next you will find a sample *SL♦ILP-S Scoring Summary Sheet* with the results of the two sample inventories as well as another rating when Jerome was in high school. It can be seen that he remembers not having too much difficulty as a child, but recalls some vivid problems related to his stuttering in high school. His stuttering is much better at his current age of thirty-two, although there are still areas of concern. The total of his scores on seven of the eight items relating to how stuttering affects or has affected him (Jerome's Total Effect Scores) for age ten, high school, and now, are 25, 40, and 20, with a possible range of 7 (least effect) to 63 (most effect).

FIGURE 1. Version to be used in rating yourself for the present time.

St. Louis Inventory of Life Perspectives and Stuttering (SL◆ILP-S)
A **Taking Stock** Self-Study Exercise • Kenneth O. St. Louis, Ph.D.

Name: _Jerome_   Age: _32_   Date: _5 - 15_

Instructions: After each of the following questions, please circle the number that best represents your opinion. Be as honest as you can. There are no right or wrong answers.

1. | Overall, how much DIFFICULTY, HANDICAP, OR SUFFERING do you experience from your stuttering *at this time.*

1	2	(3)	4	5	6	7	8	9	?
None				Moderate				Very Much	I Don't Know

2. | Overall, how much does your stuttering NEGATIVELY AFFECT YOUR ABILITY TO INTERACT WITH OTHER PEOPLE *at this time?*

1	2	(3)	4	5	6	7	8	9	?
No Negative Effect				Moderate Negative Effect				Extreme Negative Effect	I Don't Know

3. | Overall, how much do you FEEL ABLE OR UNABLE TO CONTROL YOUR STUTTERING *at this time?*

1	(2)	3	4	5	6	7	8	9	?
Completely Able to Control				Equally Able or Unable to Control				Completely Unable to Control	I Don't Know

4. | Overall, how SEVERE is your stuttering *at this time?*

1	2	(3)	4	5	6	7	8	9	?
No Stuttering	Very Mild			Moderate				Very Severe	I Don't Know

5. | Overall, how much do you FEEL A NEED OR DESIRE TO GET HELP for your stuttering *at this time?*

1	2	3	(4)	5	6	7	8	9	?
None				Moderate				Very Much	I Don't Know

6. | HOW IMPORTANT A PROBLEM IS STUTTERING IN YOUR LIFE *at this time?*

1	2	(3)	4	5	6	7	8	9	?
Not Important At All				Moderate				Very Important	I Don't Know

© Populore® 2001

7. **HOW IMPORTANT A PROBLEM IS YOUR STUTTERING IN THE LIVES OF THE PEOPLE YOU LIVE WITH** *at this time?*

1	(2)	3	4	5	6	7	8	9	?

Not Important At All   Moderate   Very Important   NA (e.g., I Live Alone) or I Don't Know

8. Overall, how much do you **FEEL INCLINED TO ASSOCIATE WITH OTHER PEOPLE WHO STUTTER** *at this time?*

1	2	3	4	5	6	7	(8)	9	?

Not At All   Moderate   Very Much   I Don't Know

9. Overall, how much do you **FEEL INCLINED TO HELP OTHER PEOPLE WHO STUTTER** *at this time?*

1	2	3	4	5	6	(7)	8	9	?

Not At All   Moderate   Very Much   I Don't Know

10. Overall, how is your **PHYSICAL HEALTH** *at this time?*

1	2	3	4	5	6	7	(8)	9	?

Very Poor   Not Poor but Not Good   Excellent   I Don't Know

11. Overall, how is your **MENTAL HEALTH** *at this time?*

1	2	3	4	5	6	7	(8)	9	?

Very Poor   Not Poor but Not Good   Excellent   I Don't Know

12. Overall, how **SATISFIED WITH YOUR LIFE** are you *at this time?*

1	2	3	4	5	6	(7)	8	9	?

Highly Unsatisfied   Not Unsatisfied but Not Satisfied   Highly Satisfied   I Don't Know

13. Overall, how much did your **STUTTERING AFFECT YOUR ANSWER ON THE PREVIOUS QUESTION, No. 12. above?**

1	(2)	3	4	5	6	7	8	9	?

No Effect on #12   Moderate Effect on #12   Completely Determined #12   I Don't Know

St. Louis Inventory of Life Perspectives and Stuttering/Recollections (SL♦ILP-S/R)
A **Taking Stock** Self-Study Exercise • Kenneth O. St. Louis, Ph.D.

Name: _Jerome_   Age: _32_   Date: _5-15_

Circle or write the the time period in the past selected for rating:

(around 10 years old)   high school   other: _____

Instructions: After each of the following questions, please circle the number that represents your current best guess of how you think you would have filled out the inventory at that time in the past indicated above. Be as honest as you can. There are no right or wrong answers.

1. | Overall, how much DIFFICULTY, HANDICAP, OR SUFFERING did you experience from your stuttering *at that time.*

| 1 | 2 | 3 | (4) | 5 | 6 | 7 | 8 | 9 | ? |

None   Moderate   Very Much   I Don't Know

2. | Overall, how much did your stuttering NEGATIVELY AFFECT YOUR ABILITY TO INTERACT WITH OTHER PEOPLE *at that time?*

| 1 | 2 | 3 | (4) | 5 | 6 | 7 | 8 | 9 | ? |

No Negative Effect   Moderate Negative Effect   Extreme Negative Effect   I Don't Know

3. | Overall, how much did you FEEL ABLE OR UNABLE TO CONTROL YOUR STUTTERING *at that time?*

| 1 | 2 | 3 | 4 | (5) | 6 | 7 | 8 | 9 | ? |

Completely Able to Control   Equally Able or Unable to Control   Completely Unable to Control   I Don't Know

4. | Overall, how SEVERE was your stuttering *at that time?*

| 1 | 2 | 3 | (4) | 5 | 6 | 7 | 8 | 9 | ? |

No Stuttering   Very Mild   Moderate   Very Severe   I Don't Know

5. | Overall, how much did you FEEL A NEED OR DESIRE TO GET HELP for your stuttering *at that time?*

| 1 | (2) | 3 | 4 | 5 | 6 | 7 | 8 | 9 | ? |

None   Moderate   Very Much   I Don't Know

6. How important a problem was stuttering in your life *at that time?*

1	2	③	4	5	6	7	8	9	?

Not Important At All — Moderate — Very Important — I Don't Know

7. How important a problem was your stuttering in the lives of the people you live with *at that time?*

①	2	3	4	5	6	7	8	9	?

Not Important At All — Moderate — Very Important — NA or I Don't Know

8. Overall, how much did you feel inclined to associate with other people who stutter *at that time?*

①	2	3	4	5	6	7	9	9	?

Not At All — Moderate — Very Much — I Don't Know

9. Overall, how much did you feel inclined to help other people who stutter *at that time?*

①	2	3	4	5	6	7	8	9	?

Not At All — Moderate — Very Much — I Don't Know

10. Overall, how was your physical health *at that time?*

1	2	3	4	5	6	7	8	⑨	?

Very Poor — Not Poor but Not Good — Excellent — I Don't Know

11. Overall, how was your mental health *at that time?*

1	2	3	4	5	6	7	8	⑨	?

Very Poor — Not Poor but Not Good — Excellent — I Don't Know

12. Overall, how satisfied with your life were you *at that time?*

1	2	3	4	5	6	7	⑧	9	?

Highly Unsatisfied — Not Unsatisfied but Not Satisfied — Highly Satisfied — I Don't Know

13. Overall, how much did your stuttering *at that time* affect your answer on the previous question, No. 12. above?

1	2	③	4	5	6	7	8	9	?

No Effect on #12 — Moderate Effect on #12 — Completely Determined #12 — I Don't Know

FIGURE 3. SL•ILP-S summary information for up to three different time periods.

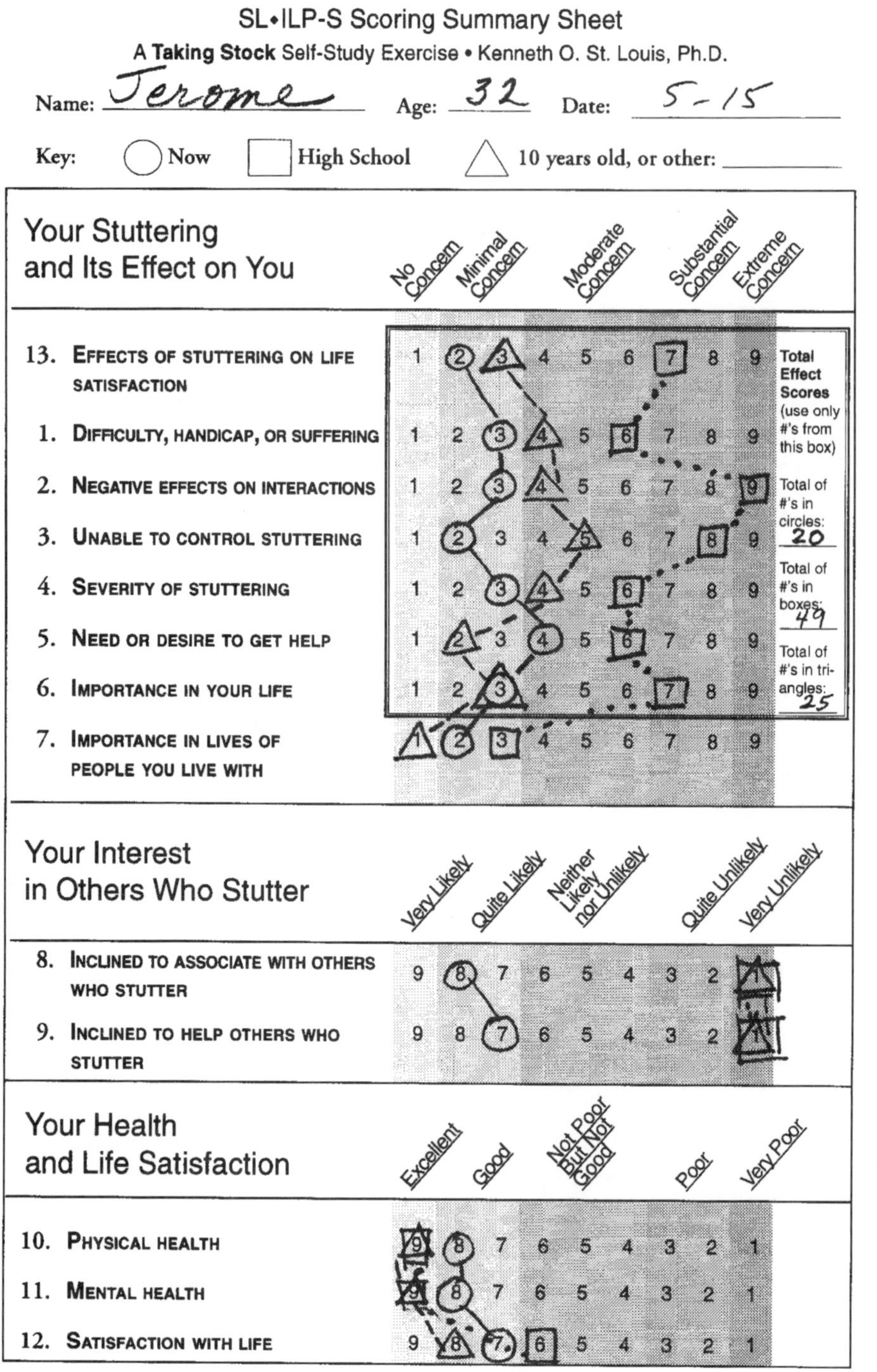

SL•ILP-S Scoring Summary Sheet
A **Taking Stock** Self-Study Exercise • Kenneth O. St. Louis, Ph.D.

Name: _Jerome_ Age: _32_ Date: _5 - 15_

Key: ◯ Now   ☐ High School   △ 10 years old, or other: _____

Your Stuttering and Its Effect on You

| | No Concern | Minimal Concern | Moderate Concern | Substantial Concern | Extreme Concern |

13. EFFECTS OF STUTTERING ON LIFE SATISFACTION   1 ② ③ 4 5 6 ☐7 8 9

1. DIFFICULTY, HANDICAP, OR SUFFERING   1 2 ③ △4 5 ☐6 7 8 9

2. NEGATIVE EFFECTS ON INTERACTIONS   1 2 ③ △4 5 6 7 8 ☐9

3. UNABLE TO CONTROL STUTTERING   1 ② 3 4 △5 6 7 ☐8 9

4. SEVERITY OF STUTTERING   1 2 ③ △4 5 ☐6 7 8 9

5. NEED OR DESIRE TO GET HELP   1 △2 3 ④ 5 ☐6 7 8 9

6. IMPORTANCE IN YOUR LIFE   1 2 ③ 4 5 6 ☐7 8 9

7. IMPORTANCE IN LIVES OF PEOPLE YOU LIVE WITH   △1 ② ☐3 4 5 6 7 8 9

Total Effect Scores (use only #'s from this box)

Total of #'s in circles: **20**

Total of #'s in boxes: **49**

Total of #'s in triangles: **25**

Your Interest in Others Who Stutter

| | Very Likely | Quite Likely | Neither Likely nor Unlikely | Quite Unlikely | Very Unlikely |

8. INCLINED TO ASSOCIATE WITH OTHERS WHO STUTTER   9 ⑧ 7 6 5 4 3 2 ☒△

9. INCLINED TO HELP OTHERS WHO STUTTER   9 8 ⑦ 6 5 4 3 2 ☒△

Your Health and Life Satisfaction

| | Excellent | Good | Not Poor But Not Good | Poor | Very Poor |

10. PHYSICAL HEALTH   ☒△9 ⑧ 7 6 5 4 3 2 1

11. MENTAL HEALTH   ☒△9 ⑧ 7 6 5 4 3 2 1

12. SATISFACTION WITH LIFE   9 △8 ⑦ ☐6 5 4 3 2 1

Some pilot data on the SL◆ILP-S.

I asked a number of speech-language pathologists around the country to assist me in gathering summary information about the *SL◆ILP-S* and mailed them questionnaires similar to the sample form provided. I also gave it to some of the clients in our Speech Clinic at West Virginia University and to a number of people whom my students had interviewed (including some featured in this book). There were 120 individuals who returned the questionnaire, most of them in Business Reply envelopes. In order to preserve anonymity, I didn't request names, but I did add a few questions about age, educational level, experience with therapy and self-help or support groups, age of onset of the stuttering, and so on.

Caution

It is important to repeat that the *SL◆ILP-S* is not what speech-language pathologists, educators, psychologists, and others refer to as a "standardized test." Such tests are used to determine the extent to which a person is normal, like an intelligence test. The *SL◆ILP-S* is, as noted above, designed strictly as a self-study exercise.

Nevertheless, I wanted to field-test the questionnaire with a fairly large group of adults who stutter to find out how they were likely to rate the various items. I also wanted to find out how similarly they rated the items as they went through the *SL◆ILP-S*. What follows is a summary of some of the information I obtained. Among other things, I included the mean (the arithmetic average), the median (the score in the middle), and the mode (the most commonly occurring score), but these should not be used to determine what is average or normal. They only describe the typical stuttering person in the field-test sample. As you look over these "measures of central tendency," remember that they don't take into account the variability of scores. For example, you might be interested to know that the range for ratings was from 1 to 9 for 11 of the 13 items, 3 to 9 for one item, and 5 to 9 for one item. If we exclude the ratings for "I don't know," of the total of 117 possible ratings (13 items *times* 9 choices), only 8 (7%) were not scored at least once by somebody.

Profile of subjects

There were 120 subjects. Of those who identified their sex, 75% were men and 25% were women. Regarding the onset or first appearance of their stuttering, 109 of the 120 adults indicated an age range as follows: before 4 years—37%; 4 to 6 years—42%; 7 to 10 years—15%; 11 to 15 years—5%, 16 to 20 years—2%. No one identified a later age of onset. The mean age of these individuals was 39.0 years with a range of 18 to 79 years. They were quite well educated on the average with a mean of 16.8 years of school (range = 10 to 28). The average number of years of speech therapy was 4.0 (range = 0 to 21 years) and self-help or support group attendance, 1.9 years (range = 0 to 15 years).

I asked about where they had lived mainly as a child. Of those who answered, 35% identified rural settings, 46% suburban settings, and 19% urban settings. Most of the questionnaires were mailed back to me in Business Reply envelopes, thirteen (11%) of which had no postmarks. Of the remainder of the subjects, twenty-one different states were represented. West Virginia was the highest with 30 subjects; followed by Colorado (13); Virginia (7); Maine, Pennsylvania, and Florida (6 each); North Carolina, Indiana, Washington DC, Alabama, and Michigan (4 each); Nebraska (3); Ohio, Maryland, New York, New Jersey, and Illinois (2 each); and Tennessee, Mississippi, Missouri, and Massachusetts (1 each).

The respondents listed a wide variety of occupations or careers as follows: attorney (2), business management (3), clergy (3), clerical (5), college professor (5), college administration (1), consultant (1), product design (2), engineer (10), financial management or service (10), government (3), graphics (1), health care (4), homemaker (3), human service (12), information management (4), media (1), natural resources (1), personnel management (4), pharmacy (1), pilot (1), recreation (1), sales (2), science (3), self business (1), skilled labor (6), student (27), teacher (8), technology (3), unskilled labor (2), and writer (1). Obviously, these subjects represent a wide range of the general population, but we cannot assume that this group is a representative sample. My guess is that more of these people attended therapy and self-help or support groups than the random stutterer in the population since they were mostly recruited by my speech-language pathology colleagues. Nevertheless, it is heartening to see that the list of occupations or careers supports the fact that stutterers can be found in virtually any field of work.

There are no right or wrong answers...

The following graphs in Figures 4 - 16 show the percentages of responses for each of the various choices on the thirteen *SL•ILP-S* items. You can easily determine the most and least common ratings for each item. Don't be concerned if your ratings do not match the common responses. Subjects ratings are for "at this time in my life." After the thirteen graphs, Table 1 shows the average scores in terms of means, medians, and modes.

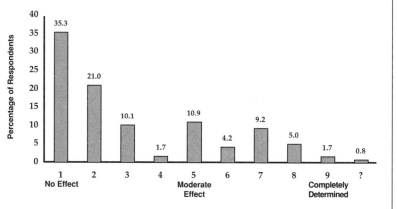

FIGURE 4. Overall, how much did your stuttering affect your rating of satisfaction with your life at this time? (#13).

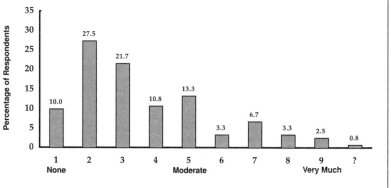

FIGURE 5. Overall, how much difficulty, handicap, or suffering do you experience from your stuttering at this time? (#1).

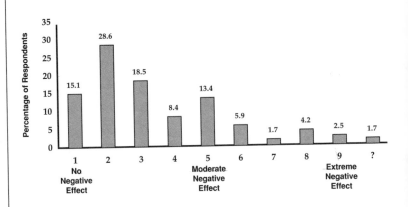

FIGURE 6. Overall, how much does your stuttering negatively affect your ability to interact with other people at this time? (#2).

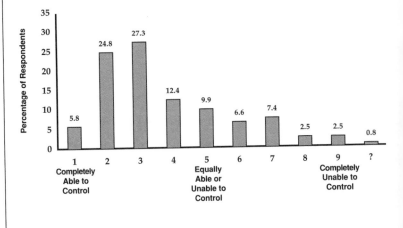

FIGURE 7. Overall, how much do you feel able or unable to control your stuttering at this time? (#3).

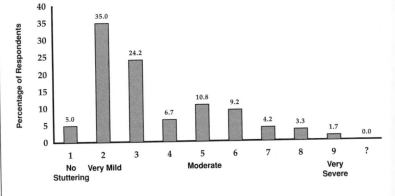

FIGURE 8. Overall, how severe is your stuttering at this time? (#4).

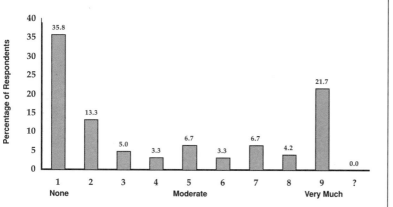

FIGURE 9. Overall, how much do you feel a need or desire to get help for your stuttering at this time? (#5).

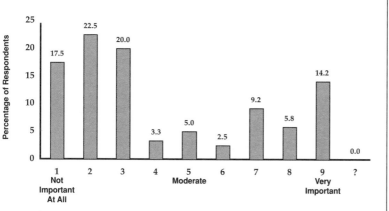

FIGURE 10. How important a problem is stuttering in your life at this time? (#6).

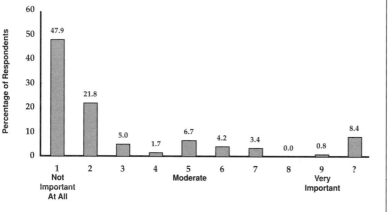

FIGURE 11. How important a problem is your stuttering in the lives of the people you live with at this time? (#7).

FIGURE 12.
Overall,
how much
do you feel
inclined to
associate
with other
people who
stutter at
this time?
(#8).

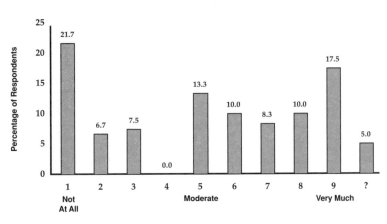

FIGURE 13
Overall,
how much
do you feel
inclined to
help other
people who
stutter at
this time?
(#9).

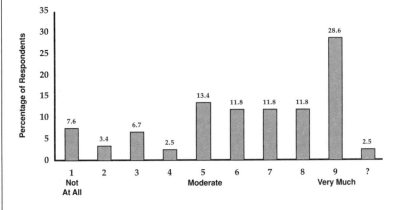

FIGURE 14.
Overall,
how is your
physical
health at
this time?
(#10).

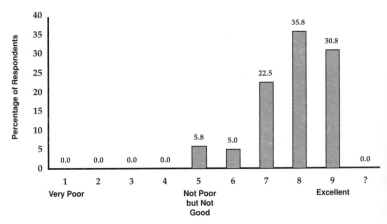

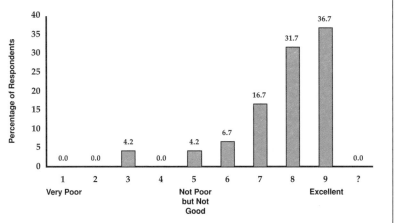

FIGURE 15. Overall, how is your mental health at this time? (#11).

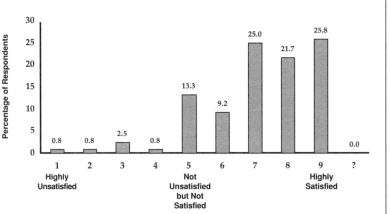

FIGURE 16. Overall, how satisfied with your life are you at this time? (#12).

Item	Mean	Median	Mode
13. Stuttering's effect on satisfaction with life	3.17	2	1
1. Difficulty, handicap, or suffering	3.59	3	2
2. Negative effect on interactions	3.38	3	2
3. Ability to control stuttering	3.73	3	3
4. Severity of stuttering	3.54	3	2
5. Desire/need for help	4.19	3	1
6. Importance in your life	4.14	3	2
7. Importance in others' lives	2.22	1	1
8. Inclined to associate with other stutters	5.05	5	1
9. Inclined to help other people who stutter	6.32	7	9
10. Physical health	7.81	8	8
11. Mental health	7.73	8	9
12. Satisfaction with life	7.16	7	9

TABLE 1. Means, medians, and modes for each of the items of the SL✦ILP-S.

Correlations

I calculated correlation coefficients (Pearson product moment) for each of the items with each of the other items and summarized them in Table 2. With the number of subjects analyzed, correlations greater than + .195 or less than -.195 are significant at the .05 level (for those who care about statistical significance). The highest correlations occurred between ratings for the amount of difficulty, suffering, or handicap experienced and the extent to which stuttering affects the ability to interact with other people (+.86). This means that high scores on one are very likely to be associated with proportionally high scores on the other, and vice versa. Also, these first two items on the *SL•ILP-S* were correlated quite strongly with several other items, that is, the ability to control stuttering, severity of stuttering, need or desire for help, the importance of stuttering in one's own life, and even the importance of stuttering in the lives of those around the stutterer. The items relating to satisfaction with one's life and the effect of stuttering on life satisfaction were moderately correlated to the above items as well.

You will note that some of the correlations are negative. This means that high ratings on one item are related to proportionally low ratings on the other. For example the respondents were quite likely to circle high ratings for satisfaction with their lives and low ratings on the amount of difficulty, handicap or suffering experienced. Also, most older subjects were more likely to give lower ratings on eight of the items on the *SL•ILP-S* than younger subjects, suggesting that stuttering does tend to get better over time.

There was no significant correlation between a person's likelihood of associating with another stutterer or his or her likelihood of helping another stutterer and any of the other items, but these two items were strongly correlated with each other. Interestingly, mental health was weakly to moderately correlated with most of the other items. It was also correlated with physical health, but ratings for physical heath had lower correlations than the ratings for mental health. Except for two very low significant results, the age of onset of stuttering was not correlated with any of the other items. There was a moderate negative correlation between life satisfaction and the effects of stuttering on satisfaction. This means that the more satisfied one was with his or her life, the less effect stuttering had on that rating. Yet, in spite of the -.52 correlation here, there were a few interesting exceptions in the questionnaire choices. A few subjects

	1	2	3	4	5	6	7	8	9	10	11	12	13	14	15
1. Difficulty, handicap, suffering	—														
2. Negative effect on interactions	0.86*	—													
3. Ability to control stuttering	0.65*	0.60*	—												
4. Severity of stuttering	0.75*	0.72*	0.80*	—											
5. Desire/ need for help	0.66*	0.66*	0.47*	0.64*	—										
6. Importance in your life	0.75*	0.78*	0.50*	0.66*	0.80*	—									
7. Importance in others' lives	0.58*	0.60*	0.40*	0.53*	0.54*	0.65*	—								
8. Inclined to associate with other stutters	0.09	0.10	0.08	0.11	0.18	0.11	0.05	—							
9. Inclined to help others who stutter	0.04	0.09	0.03	0.04	0.15	0.09	0.04	0.60*	—						
10. Physical health	-0.21*	-0.21*	-0.17	-0.15	0.01	-0.03	-0.07	0.01	-0.02	—					
11. Mental health	-0.50*	-0.52*	-0.27*	-0.29*	0.24*	-0.33*	-0.31*	-0.10	-0.01	0.52*	—				
12. Life satisfaction	-0.54*	-0.58*	-0.44*	-0.43*	0.33*	-0.47*	-0.48*	-0.11	-0.04	0.29*	-0.59*	—			
13. Life and stuttering	0.55*	0.65*	0.38*	0.54*	0.50*	0.61*	0.47*	0.04	0.13	-0.12	0.23*	0.52*	—		
14. Onset	-0.09	-0.02	-0.05	-0.09	0.05	0.01	-0.20*	-0.09	-0.12	0.08	0.21	0.17	0.08	—	
15. Age	-0.35*	-0.26*	-0.14	-0.21*	0.31*	-0.42*	-0.26*	-0.05	0.16	0.25*	0.08	0.20*	-0.10	0.00	—

TABLE 2. Correlations for 15 SL♦ILP-S items.

* $r > \pm .195$ at $p < .05$

scored both items high, that is, they were very satisfied with their lives *and* they indicated that stuttering played a major role in that satisfaction.

Finally, the results for the Total Effect Score are shown below in the last graph. I calculated all the Total Effect Scores for the 120 subjects, sorted them from lowest to highest, and then plotted them in Figure 17. Since there are seven items, the possible scores range from 0 to 63 (7 times 9). "I don't know" ratings are not counted in the total. You can see that the 120 stutterers had Total Effect Scores ranging from 5 to 59 which indicates that they ranged from totally free of any difficulty from stuttering to severely affected. The mean was 25.6, the median was 22.5, and the mode was 12. If the scores are divided by 7s, 3% were 7 and below, 27% between 8 and 14, 17% between 15 and 21, 18% between 22 and 28, 10% between 29 and 35, 5% between 36 and 42, 13% between 43 and 49, 5% between 50 and 56, and 2% over 57. In general, the Total Effect Score would be expected to drop as a person became more and more accepting of—and unaffected by—his or her stuttering.

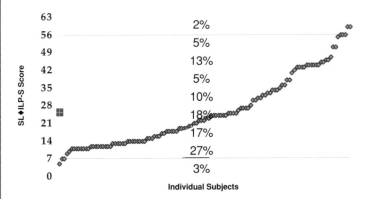

FIGURE 17. Scores for individual subjects on seven *SL♦ILP-S* items pertaining to the effects of stuttering on one's life.

♦ Individual Total Effect Score
⊞ Mean of 120 Total Effect Scores

Name Index

A

Ahlbach, J. 7, 8, 19, 25, 179, 200
Ambrose, N. 142
Aronson, A. 218

B

Baker, M. 24, 65
Bakker, K. 8
Barrett, R. 199
Baumeister, R. 179
Baumgartner, J. 179
Bedford, K. 8
Benson, V. 19, 179
Bernstein Ratner, N. 142, 179, 180, 181, 189
Blood, G. 148, 179, 199, 211
Bloodstein, O. 150, 153, 179, 192, 218
Bloom, C. 179
Boberg, E. 8
Bondarenko, V. 185, 188, 191
Bossart, G. 8
Bosshardt, H-G. 148, 183
Boyd, L. 8
Brown, S. 218
Brutten, G. 8, 143, 180

C

Caggiano, L. 185, 188
Caseman, L. 25, 119
Caudill, A. 8
Chesterton, G. 7
Chmela, K. 179, 185
Cilek, T. 200
Clinton, W. 68
Coleman Carpenter, M. 24, 103
Conture, E. 179, 191
Cook, F. 187
Cooper, C. 211
Cooper, E. 8, 218
Cooperman, D. 179
Cordes, A. 180
Corley, V. 24, 61
Costello, J. 165, 179
Costine, B. 25, 123
Cox, M. 179
Creaghead, N. 211
Crocket, K. 20, 181
Curlee, R. 8, 143, 144, 150, 151, 179, 180, 182, 189, 192, 218
Curtis, J. 218

D

Daly, D. 8, 180
Davis, J. 24, 110
Davis, L. 218
Dayton, R. 187, 190
De Geus, E. 189
De Nil, L. 180, 188
Demosthenes 157
Densmore, A. 199
Diaz, C. 189
Diggs, C. 148, 183, 185, 188
Digrande, A. 198
Doan, R. 20, 21, 181
Donaher, J. 190
Durrenberger, C. 182

E

Edney, C. 218
Eisenson, J. 139, 180
Epston, D. 20, 181, 183, 219

F

Ferketic, M. 211
Ferree, H. 8
Frankl, V. 19, 180
Fraser, J. 185, 193, 203
Fraser, M. 203
Frederick, M. 8
Freund, H. 180
Fry, J. 187

G

Georgieva, D. 8
Givens-Ackerman, J. 182
Glenn, A. 160
Glenn, J. 160
Goebel, M. 180, 198
Goldberg, L. 211
Gooden, R. 21
Gray, D. 24, 69
Gregory, H. 8, 211
Guitar, B. 155, 160, 180, 191, 218
Gurrister, T. 199

H

Hacker, K. 23, 39
Hall, F. 187
Ham, R. 180
Hanley, J. 211
Hanna, J. 24, 106
Haroldson, S. 180, 181, 218

Harrison

Harrison, F. 25, 127
Harrison, J. 189
Healey, E. C. 147, 180, 181, 185
Helekar, S. 189
Helm-Estabrooks, N. 150, 180, 218
Hicks, R. 186, 189
Hightower, C. 8, 22, 210
Hillis, J. 180
Hoagland, E. 180
Hollingdale, R. 181
Honig, C. 8
Hood, S. 140, 182, 185, 211
Hriblan, L. 187, 190
Hughes, M. 186, 189

I

Ingham, R. 180
Inskeep, E. 121

J

Jaffe, A. 23, 41
Janssen, P. 143, 180
Jezer, M. 19, 180, 185, 186, 190
Johnson, A. 206
Johnson, W. 139, 152-153, 180, 218
Johnston, G. 185
Jones, J. 46-48
Jones, K. 199

K

Kathard, H. 188
Keaster, J. 218
Kelly, E. 151, 182
Kloth, S. 143, 180
Kolk, H. 180, 218
Kraaimaat, F. 143, 180
Krieger, K. 199
Kroll, R. 199
Kuhl, P. 181
Kully-Martens, D. 198
Kuster, J. 184, 188, 191, 197, 203

L

Langevin, M. 147, 181
Lass, N. 8, 182
Lee, S. 24, 99
Leith, W. 8
Lennex, K. 8
Lew, G. 189, 190
Lewis, F. 23, 57
Lewis, K. 186, 190
Lincoln, M. 189

Note

Individuals whose names are in bold are authors of one of the stories in Chapter 2.

Lubker, B. 8, 148, 183
Lundeen, C. 144, 182

M

Maansson, H. 190
Mandler, J. 17, 181
Manning, W. 167, 181, 185, 186, 189, 192
Martin, R. 8, 180, 181, 218
McDonald, J. 8
McPherson, C. 200
Meyer, R. 180
Monk, G. 20, 181
Moses 144
Mowrer, D. 204
Murphy, B. 181, 187, 190
Murray, F. 18, 181
Myers, F. 8, 144, 160, 181, 182, 183, 189

N

Natke, U. 189
Neiders, G. 186, 190
Neilson, M. 8
Newman, L. 179
Nietzsche, F. 19, 181
Niner, P. 24, 116
Norris, J. 185
Novotny, A. 8

O

Oakes, K. 8
Onslow, M. 155, 181
Otto Montgomery, C. 198

P

Padgett, L. 24, 88
Parry, A. 20, 21, 181
Parry, W. 184, 186
Pavlov 154
Perkins, W. 165, 179, 182, 218
Peters, H. 8, 147, 148, 181, 183
Peters, T. 211, 218
Phillips, C. 187, 190
Pill, J. 8, 148, 183

Postma, A. 180, 218
Power, M. 199
Pratt, H. 25, 131
Preece, D. 186, 189
Progoff, I. 181, 224
Purser, H. 170, 182

Q

Quesal, R. 8, 24, 73, 181, 185, 186, 188, 189, 203

R

Rainer, T. 25, 181
Ratner, N. See Bernstein Ratner
Reardon, N. 179
Reeves, L. 171, 181, 186, 188, 190
Robinson, B. 218
Roden, L. 186, 190
Rosenfield, D. 189
Ross, D. 199
Roth, C. 218
Rowley, D. 170, 182
Ruscello, D. 8, 144, 182
Rustin, L. 8, 170, 182
Ryan, B. 165, 182

S

Schiffbauer, J. 187, 190
Scott Trautman, L. 185
Sedlock, A. 187, 190
Shapiro, D. 167, 168, 182, 192
Sheehan, J. 54-57, 82-88, 182
Siegel, G. 144, 151, 164, 180, 182, 192, 218
Sielen, R. J. 7
Silverman, E-M. 189
Sliger, A. 24, 77
Smith, A. 151, 182
Snyder, G. 23, 45
Sobel, R. 182
St. Louis, E. 7
St. Louis, D. 8
St. Louis, K. 24, 94, 140, 144, 148, 170, 181, 182, 183, 184, 187, 189, 190, 211, 218

St. Louis, M. 7, 183
St. Louis, R. 8
Starke, A. 186
Starkweather, C. W. 8, 182, 186, 189, 198, 204, 211, 218
Starr, C. 180
Steiner, D. 186, 190
Sturm, B. 23, 53
Sugarman, M. 8, 24, 81, 186, 206
Summerlin, T. 23, 35
Susca, M. 185

T

Taffoni, M. 8
Thomas, J. 25, 135
Travis, L. 183
Triden, K. 218

V

Van Der Berg, A. 186, 190
Van Riper, C. 54-57, 139, 161, 162, 165, 167, 183, 218
Viswanath, N. 189

W

Wall, M. 160, 183
Wallace, M. 183
Walton, P. 183
Webster, R. 183, 199
Weiner, H. 189
Westbrook, J. 170, 182, 211
White, M. 17, 20, 183, 219
Williams, D. 189
Wilson, M. 23, 48
Wingate, M. 218
Winslade, J. 20, 181

Y

Yairi, E. 143, 180
Yaruss, J. S. 8, 148, 183

Z

Zebrowski, P. 142, 183, 200

Topic Index

A

Acceptance 46–48, 62–65, 82–88, 100–103, 111–116, 120–123
Accessory behaviors 70–73, 78–81, 95–99, 144, 146, 154, 216. *See also* Stuttering: Symptoms; Terminology
American Institute for Stuttering 198
American Speech-Language-Hearing Association (ASHA) 172, 201
Anger. *See* Emotions
Annandale Fluency Clinic, Inc. 198
Anticipation 36–39, 49–53, 95–99
Anxiety. *See* Emotions
Approach-avoidance conflict 82–88
Articulation errors 46–48, 111–116, 120–123, 143
ASHA. *See* American Speech-Language-Hearing Association

B

Behavior modification. *See* Cause: Operant conditioning; Speech therapy approaches: Contingent management
Bill of Rights and Responsibilities for People who Stutter 205–206
Birch Tree Foundation 198
Blocks. *See* Stuttering: Symptoms. *See also* Terminology
Board Recognized Specialist in Fluency Disorders 196
Books (recommended)
For adults who stutter 184–187
For new SLP students 187–190
For the general public 187–190
For trained SLPs 190–193
Boston University 198
Brochures (recommended)
For adults who stutter 184–187
For new SLP students 187–190
For the general public 187–190
For trained SLPs 190–193

C

Canadian Association for People Who Stutter (CAPS) 200
Canadian Association of Speech-Language Pathologists and Audiologists (CASLPA) 202
Cancellation. *See* Speech therapy approaches: Stuttering modification
Career. *See* Effects on life

CASLPA. *See* Canadian Association of Speech-Language Pathologists and Audiologists
Cause 148–155
Classical conditioning 154
Combination of factors 49–53, 66–69, 128–131
Fear 54–57
Freudian influences 151
Heredity 142–143
Imitation 153
Language-based 70–73
Learning 153–155
Neurogenic 23, 150
Neuromotor problems 70–73, 149–150
Neurosis 151
Operant conditioning 155
Physical problems 40–41, 62–65
Physiological problems 149–150
Psychogenic 153, 218
Psychological problems 70–73, 151–153
Punishment 117–119
Talking fast 66–69
Teasing 95–99
Trauma 49–53
CCC/SLP. *See* Certificate of Clinical Competence
Certificate of Clinical Competence (CCC/SLP) 172, 195
Chronic stuttering 141
Classical conditioning. *See* Cause
Clearinghouses on stuttering 203
Clinic. *See* Speech therapy
Cluttering 24, 143, 217
Code of Ethics (ASHA) 197
Coexisting problems 143–144
Columbia Speech and Language Services 198
Comprehensive Stuttering Program 198
Contingent management. *See* Speech therapy approaches
Core behaviors 70–73. *See also* Stuttering: Symptoms
Counselor 132–135
Courses in stuttering 172
Credentials. *See* Board Recognized Specialist in Fluency Disorders; Certificate of Clinical Competence

D

DAF *See* Delayed auditory feedback
Dating. *See* Effects on life

Delayed auditory feedback (DAF). *See* Speech therapy approaches: Fluency shaping
Desensitization. *See* Speech therapy approaches
Disfluencies 146. *See also* Stuttering: Symptoms
Disfluency 212. *See also* Terminology
Drug therapy 111–116
Dysfluency 213. *See also* Stuttering; Terminology

E

Effects on life 145, 176
Age 246
Career 31–35, 58–61, 62–65, 66–69, 70–73, 78–81, 89–94, 95–99, 107–110, 111–116, 124–127, 132–135, 241
Dating 89–94, 117–119
Education 31–35, 54–57, 58–61, 62–65, 66–69, 70–73, 74–77, 78–81, 117–119, 124–127, 132–135
Empathy toward others 49–53, 58–61, 74–77, 100–103, 124–127, 128–131, 244
Friends 62–65, 107–110
General outlook 42–45, 117–119, 245
Life satisfaction 31–35, 78–81, 107–110, 241, 243, 245, 246. *See also* Life perspectives and stuttering
Personality 42–45, 58–61, 62–65, 70–73, 74–77, 78–81, 82–88, 100–103, 107–110
Social life 54–57, 66–69, 70–73, 74–77, 107–110, 242
Effort 216
Embarrassment. *See* Emotions
Emotions 147
Anger 49–53, 100–103, 120–123
Anxiety 40–41, 46–48, 78–81, 82–88, 89–94, 100–103, 107–110, 120–123, 124–127
Awkwardness 70–73
Courage 117–119
Determination 117–119
Embarrassment 31–35, 40–41, 49–53, 66–69, 70–73, 82–88, 100–103, 111–116, 124–127
Envy 95–99
Fear 31–35, 46–48, 58–61, 70–73, 78–81, 100–103, 104–106, 117–119

Note

The page numbers for entries referring to a topic covered in one of the Chapter 2 stories are given in bold. For these, a page *range* is given. The range is for the entire story; the topic is covered somewhere within that range.

Emotions (continued)
  Frustration 40–41, 74–77, 82–88,
    120–123, 128–131
  Guilt 31–35, 42–45, 78–81
  Hope 82–88, 117–119
  Optimism 36–39, 40–41, 82–88,
    117–119, 175
  Pessimism 117–119
  Rejection 128–131
  Shame 31–35, 42–45, 78–81,
    82–88
Epidemiology. *See* Stuttering:
    Incidence; Stuttering:
    Prevalence
Evaluation 66–69
Expectancy. *See* Anticipation

F

False-role disorder 82–88
Fear. *See* Emotions: Anxiety;
    Emotions: Fear
Fluency 212. *See also* Terminology
Fluency disorder 140, 212. *See*
    Cluttering; Stuttering. *See also*
    Terminology
Fluency Intensive Center for
    Communication Disorders
    199
Fluency shaping. *See* Speech therapy
    approaches
Friends 200
Frustration. *See* Emotions

G

Gender 141–142. *See also* Stuttering:
    Incidence; Stuttering:
    Prevalence
Genetics. *See* Cause: Heredity
Goals
  Acceptance of stuttering 31–35,
    49–53, 70–73, 74–77, 82–88,
    132–135
  Become effective communicator
    54–57
  Consistent fluency 82–88
  Get education 95–99, 100–103
  Help others 54–57, 89–94
  Overcome negative emotions
    31–35, 66–69, 70–73, 82–88,
    95–99, 117–119. *See also*
    Emotions
  Recovery 31–35, 49–53, 82–88,
    95–99, 100–103, 120–123,
    128–131
  Stutter less 40–41, 100–103,
    117–119. *See also* Recovery

H

Harold B. Starbuck Memorial Fluency
    Enhancing Clinics 199
Health
  Mental 245, 246
  Physical 244

Helpers (miscellaneous). *See* Speech
    therapy approaches
Heredity. *See* Cause
Hollins Fluency System 199
Hope. *See* Emotions

I

IALP. *See* International Association of
    Logopedics and Phoniatrics
IFA. *See* International Fluency
    Association
Incidence. *See* Stuttering
Indiana University/Sertoma Speech
    Camp 199
Instrumental conditioning 154. *See
    also* Cause: Operant
    conditioning
International Association of
    Logopedics and Phoniatrics
    (IALP) 202
International Fluency Association
    (IFA) 203
International Stuttering Association
    (ISA) 201
International Stuttering Awareness
    Day (ISAD) 204
International stuttering research
    institute 89–94
Internet resources (recommended)
    203–204
  For adults who stutter 184–187
  For new SLP students 187–190
  For the general public 187–190
  For trained SLPs 190–193
Interview
  Benefits 22
  Tape recording 222–223
  Tips 222–223
ISA. *See* International Stuttering
    Association
ISAD. *See* International Stuttering
    Awareness Day

J

Jobs. *See* Effects on life: Career
Journaling 224

L

Language problems 143
Life perspectives and stuttering
    231–248
Linguistic hierarchy management. *See*
    Speech therapy approaches
Logotherapy 19
Low self-esteem 49–53, 62–65,
    95–99, 100–103, 128–131

M

Maintenance 74–77, 89–94. *See also*
    Speech therapy approaches
Memoirs 18

N

Narrative psychology 17
Narrative therapy 19, 20, 220
National Stuttering Association (NSA)
    54–57, 78–81, 89–94, 170,
    174, 200
Naturalness 217
Neurogenic stuttering 217 *See also*
    Cause
Never give up. *See* Emotions:
    Determination
Non-standardized test 239
NSA. *See* National Stuttering
    Association

O

On-line conferences. *See* International
    Stuttering Awareness Day
Onset 70–73, 132–135, 141
  Sudden onset 40–41
Operant conditioning. *See* Cause
Oral history 18
Organizations
  Professional 201–203
Other stutterers 54–57, 62–65,
    89–94, 111–116, 124–127

P

Parents 167, 152
  Attitudes 31–35, 46–48, 62–65
  Reactions 36–39, 46–48, 62–65,
    70–73, 78–81, 82–88, 89–94,
    124–127
Pennsylvania State University 199
Perfectionism 100–103, 132–135
Person-first labels 17, 26
Personal history 18
Physiological problems. *See* Cause
Postmodern therapy 20
Power Stuttering Center 199
Precision Fluency Shaping Program
    199
Predictability of stuttering 145
Prevalence. *See* Stuttering
Progression of stuttering 144–145
Prolongations. *See* Stuttering:
    Symptoms. *See also*
    Terminology
Prosody 217
Provincial associations 202. *See also*
    State associations
Psychiatrist 82–88
Psychogenic stuttering. *See* Cause
Psychological problems. *See* Cause
Psychologist 78–81
Public speaking. *See* Self-therapy: Give
    speeches

R

Rate 216. *See also* Speaking rate
Reactions to stuttering
  Another stutterer 111–116

Others' reactions 31–35, 42–45, 46–48, 49–53, 62–65, 74–77, 78–81, 100–103, 120–123, 124–127, 128–131
Parent. *See* Parent reactions
Recovery 124–127, 128–131
Regression. *See* Relapse
Relapse 74–77, 89–94
Repetitions of sounds or syllables. *See* Stuttering: Symptoms. *See also* Terminology
Research on stuttering 89–94
Respondent conditioning. *See* Cause: Classical conditioning
Rhythm 217

S

Saying own name 36–39
SBFD. *See* Specialty Board on Fluency Disorders
School. *See* Speech therapy
Secondary mannerisms. *See* Accessory behaviors. *See also* Terminology
Self-help 78–81, 89–94, 111–116, 170–171, 173, 200–201, 240, 244
Self-role conflict 82–88
Self-therapy 23, 155–157
Build confidence 31–35, 62–65, 66–69, 82–88, 95–99, 104–106, 128–131, 156, 175
Educate self on stuttering 78–81, 117–119, 132–135
Enter difficult situations 31–35, 66–69, 100–103, 117–119, 156
Get mad 157
Give speeches 31–35, 58–61, 66–69, 95–99, 124–127
Have others monitor speech 40–41
Monitor speech 36–39, 46–48, 124–127
Never give up. *See* Emotions: Determination
Pause before speaking 49–53, 58–61, 124–127, 156
Practice speaking alone 36–39, 58–61, 82–88, 132–135, 156
Preparation 95–99, 132–135
Read aloud 128–131, 156
Singing 107–110, 128–131, 156
"Sink or swim" 104–106
Skip the word 36–39
Slow down speech 40–41, 156
Spell the word 36–39
Substitute an easier word 31–35, 49–53, 66–69, 70–73, 78–81, 95–99, 111–116, 124–127, 157
Take a deep breath before speaking 31–35, 156
Talk openly about stuttering 49–53, 100–103, 124–127
Talk with pebbles in mouth 157

Tell others you stutter 31–35, 78–81, 111–116, 156
Summon the will not to stutter 128–131, 156
Use gestures to speak 78–81
Use humor 36–39, 62–65, 156, 175
Use new voice 58–61, 78–81, 107–110, 174
SFA. *See* Stuttering Foundation of America
SID 4. *See* Special Interest Division 4 on Fluency and Fluency Disorders
SL♦ILP-S. *See also* Life perspectives and stuttering
About 231–248
Form 234–235
Scoring Summary Sheet 231–233, 238
Summary data 240–248
Correlations 246–248
Negative 246
Mean 239, 245
Median 239, 245
Mode 239, 245
Total Effect Score 232, 248
SL♦ILP-S/R
About 231–232
Form 236–237
SLP. *See* Speech-Language Pathologist
SLP students 54–57, 74–77, 82–88, 111–116, 171–173
Speak Easy Inc. of Canada 201
"Speak more fluently". *See* Speech therapy approaches: Fluency shaping
Speaking rate. *See* Cause: Talking fast; Rate; Self-therapy: Slow down speech; Speech therapy approaches: Fluency shaping: Talking slower
Special Interest Division 4 on Fluency and Fluency Disorders 173, 201
Specialists 171–173, 174
Specialty Board on Fluency Disorders (SBFD) 173, 196, 202
Speech Foundation of Ontario 199
Speech-Language Pathologist (SLP) 42–45, 70–73, 82–88, 111–116
Qualifications 195–197
Speech therapist/clinician. *See* Speech-Language Pathologist
Speech therapy 70–73, 74–77, 89–94, 240, 243
Clinic 54–57, 70–73, 74–77, 78–81, 82–88, 89–94, 100–103, 120–123, 169
Effective 49–53, 54–57, 78–81, 82–88, 100–103, 120–123
Extended model 169–170
Ineffective 42–45, 49–53, 54–57, 78–81, 82–88, 89–94, 100–103, 111–116, 117–119, 120–123

Intensive model 54–57, 89–94, 169, 170, 198–200
School 46–48, 49–53, 66–69, 70–73, 78–81, 89–94, 100–103, 111–116, 117–119, 120–123, 169
Speech therapy approaches 18, 158–170
Articulation therapy 49–53, 78–81
Contingent management 42–45, 162–164
"Highlighting" hypothesis 162
Operant "punishment" 163
Time-out 163
Delayed auditory feedback (DAF). *See* Speech therapy approaches: Fluency shaping
Desensitization 165–167
Confronting fears 70–73, 78–81, 166
Counseling 78–81, 166
Entering difficult situations 82–88, 111–116, 166
Stuttering openly 54–57
Reducing avoidance 54–57, 82–88
Stuttering on purpose 54–57, 82–88, 89–94, 166
Fluency shaping 42–45, 82–88, 159–160
Correct breathing 54–57, 66–69, 111–116, 120–123, 159
Delayed auditory feedback (DAF) 159
Easy onset 111–116, 120–123, 159
Monitoring speech 78–81, 159
Real-time acoustic feedback 159
Talking slower 46–48, 159
Group discussion 54–57, 74–77, 78–81, 89–94, 111–116
Linguistic hierarchy management (progressing from easy to hard utterances) 164–165
Maintenance 168
Passive airflow 54–57
Practice in real life 89–94
Reading aloud 49–53, 78–81, 82–88
Relaxation based 54–57
Repeating phrases 70–73
Stuttering modification 54–57, 161–162
Cancellation 89–94, 161
Preparatory sets 161
Pull-outs 89–94, 161
Transfer 168
Speeches
Giving 104–106. *See also* Self-therapy: Give speeches
Spontaneous recovery 54–57, 141

St. Louis Inventory of Life Perspectives and Stuttering. *See SL◆ILP-S; SL◆ILP-S/R*
Stammering 215. *See also* Terminology
State associations 202. *See also* Provincial associations
Stereotypes 22, **31–35, 36–39, 42–45, 95–99,** 148
Stigma. *See* Stereotypes
Stories of stuttering
　Change over time 21, 219
　"Dominant" 220
　Healing 19
　Hearing 17, 19, 222
　Meaning 18
　Narrative. *See* Narrative psychology; Narrative therapy
　"Nuclear episodes" 17
　Preserving 18, 223
　"Re-visions" 20, 220
　Sharing 25
　Summary of experiences 17, 20–21
　Tape recording 222–223
　Telling 17, 19, 176, 219
　　Group 221. *See also* Speech therapy approaches: Group discussion; Support group
　　Personal interview 220–221
　　Tips 225, 227
　　To oneself 222
　Themes 21, 23–25
　Unique 20
　Writing 223
STUT-HLP 203
STUTT-L 204
STUTT-X 204

"Stutter more fluently". *See* Speech therapy approaches: Stuttering modification
Stuttering. *See also* Terminology
　Definition 139–140, 213
　Incidence 141
　Prevalence 141
　Severity 242
　Societal expectations 219
　Symptoms
　　Blocks **42–45, 70–73, 78–81, 82–88, 111–116, 120–123, 132–135**
　　Pauses **49–53, 58–61,** 104–106, 132–135
　　Prolongations 146
　　Repetition of sounds or syllables **82–88, 95–99, 111–116,** 146
Stuttering Foundation of America (SFA) 174, 196, 203
Stuttering Homepage 197, 200, 203
Stuttering modification. *See* Speech therapy approaches
Successful Stuttering Management Program 199
Summer Remedial Clinic 200
Support group 170. *See also* Self-help; Speech therapy approaches: Group discussion
Suprasegmental features 216

T

Taking stock 176, 194, 219–230, 231–238. *See also* Life perspectives and stuttering

Teasing **100–103, 124–127,** 147. *See also* Emotions
Telephone use 74–77, **89–94, 100–103,** 107–110, **124–127.** *See also* Emotions
Tension **36–39, 58–61.** *See also* Emotions
Terminology 211–218
Therapy. *See also* Self-therapy
　Approaches. *See* Speech therapy approaches
　Evaluation 222
　Seeking 195–197
　Self. *See* Self-therapy
　Transfer. *See* Speech therapy approaches

U

Universal stuttering 144

V

Videos (recommended)
　For adults who stutter 184–187
　For new SLP students 187–190
　For the general public 187–190
　For trained SLPs 190–193

W

Wendell Johnson Speech and Hearing Clinic 200

ORDER FORM

Living with Stuttering: Stories, Basics, Resources, and Hope and *Taking Stock* materials, designed especially for people who stutter, clinicians, student projects, and self-help groups.

Clip or copy this form. Please call for Canadian prices.

Telephone orders: Toll free: 866-667-8679

Postal orders: Populore Publishing Company, PO Box 4382, Morgantown, WV 26504, 304-599-3830

Fax orders: 304-599-7224

Please send me:

❑ ____ copies of *Living with Stuttering: Stories, Basics, Resources, and Hope* at $19.95 each. Shipping and handling: $4.00 for the first book ($23.95) and $2.00 for each additional book (#T1).
Total including shipping and handling: $ _____

Taking Stock: Telling Your Story Worksheet (8.5 x 11, 4 pages), includes shipping and handling.
❑ 1 copy: $3:00 (#T4)
❑ 5 copies: $8.00 (#T5)
❑ 25 copies: $20.00 (#T6)
Total: $ _____

Taking Stock: St. Louis Inventory of Life Perspectives and Stuttering (SL♦ILP-S) and the *SL♦ILP-S Summary Scoring Sheet* (8.5 x 11, 3 pages), includes shipping and handling.
❑ 1 copy of each: $3.00 (#T7)
❑ 5 copies of each: $8.00 (#T8)
❑ 25 copies of each: $20.00 (#T9)
Total: $ _____

Taking Stock: St. Louis Inventory of Life Perspectives and Stuttering/ Recollections (SL♦ILP-S/R) (for two recollection ratings per person) (8.5 x 11, 4 pages), includes shipping and handling.
❑ 2 copies: $3.00 (#T10)
❑ 10 copies $8.00 (#T11)
❑ 50 copies $20.00 (#T12)
Total: $ _____

❑ *Taking Stock Clinical or Support Group Kit* (includes 25 *Telling Your Story Worksheets*, #T6; 25 *SL♦ILP-S* questionnaires and 25 *SL♦ILP-S Summary Scoring Sheets*, #T9; and 50 *SL-ILP-S/R* questionnaires, #T12). Kit: $35.00 (#T3). ($25 savings), includes shipping and handling.
Total: $ _____

❑ *Complete Living with Stuttering Clinical or Support Group Kit* (includes 1 copy of *Living with Stuttering: Stories, Basics, Resources, and Hope*, #T1; and 1 *Taking Stock Clinical or Support Group Kit*, #T3). Kit: $50 (#T2). ($33.95 savings), includes shipping and handling.
Total: $ _____

❑ Description of products and services related to telling and preserving or publishing your own story with Populore (free).

Subtotal (add totals above) $ _____

Please add 6% sales tax for books shipped to West Virginia
(Subtotal x 0.06) $ _____

Total Payment $ _____

Ship to:

Name: _____

Full mailing address: _____

_____

_____

Phone: _____

If you wish, please tell us about yourself:

❑ I am a person who stutters.
❑ I am a family member or friend of a person who stutters.
❑ I am a Speech-Language Pathologist.
❑ Other: _____

Payment:

❑ Check (payable to Populore)

❑ Credit card: ❑ VISA   ❑ MasterCard

Card number: _____

Name printed on card: _____

Signature: _____ Exp. date: _____ / _____

Allow 2-3 weeks for delivery.

Please contact Populore (toll free: 866-667-8679) regarding additional costs or savings for Canadian sales, priority or overnight delivery, shipping to other countries, desired quantities not listed above, other quantity discounts, review copies, or desk copies for college teachers.